# the baby:

# life cycle
# of a kingdom vision

## david a. yeazell

**ISBN:** 1-4196-3715-0

**cover design and interior formatting:** Stallworth Illustrations, Grand Prairie, Texas

**photo credits:** (c) Alice De Haven, Phil Date, Isabel Poulin, Simone Van Den Berg, Jodi Hutchison, Lorelyn Medina, Les Beyerly, Tanya Weliky, Fred Goldstein and Daniela Spyropoulou; agency: Dreamstime

**editing:** Lisa Bryant, Priscilla Aikens and William Nolan

# table of contents

intimacy with Him
the soul's retreat
a visitation
now I lay me down
a bed of trust

be it unto me
God doesn't practice birth control
the master's desire
a heart's cry
stripping of reliance on the flesh

the morning after
a proper diet
controlled outside influences
a pondering heart

the labor process—long nights and warfare
the labor pains and travail
the mid-wife
the place of the birth

nanny 911
preparation of the nursery
nutrition and sanitation
disease and health

# acknowledgments

This book is first dedicated to all those unsung heroes who have spent sleepless nights in restless prayer; not fully understanding the purposes of God in their lives, but believing that there was a precious cargo in their belly that had world-changing potential. To all you and the priceless, yet personally costly, purpose that God has entrusted you to carry—God bless!

———————————————————————

To my parents, Gene and Carol Yeazell, and my sister and brother-In-law, Ernie and Melody Hays—all ministers of the Gospel and people of influence in the Kingdom, and in my personal kingdom—all my love to you!

To Pastor Vanessa Weatherspoon of Dallas; Pastor Helga Clark of Miami and Apostle Linda Evans of Brooklyn; all great mothers in the Kingdom, who told me I had a book inside waiting to be birthed—thanks for timely, prophetic encouragement to write what you saw gestating in my belly.

To some of the numerous "midwives" who encouraged me as I wrote: William Nolan, Priscilla Aikens, Elaine Robinson, Gene Little, Navolia Bryant, Janine Simpson, Thomas Henley and Ted Williams—thanks for cheering me on and pushing me forward!

To the great wordsmith, and my pastor, Bishop T.D. Jakes and his wife, Serita; thanks for all that you deposited in me over the years. You quickened the gifts inside me through assignments, both great and ordinary, and allowed me to spread my wings and fly with vision in your house—I am truly grateful!

To my countless friends, from decades of youthful and middle-aged vision and holy passion—you know who you are and where you are—remember that our wrinkles are never too deep nor our spiritual wombs too dry for Him to plant fresh seed of purpose and Kingdom defining influence in us. We may age and gray on the outside, but our inner man is being renewed daily, and may we never cease to be a channel of His vision and purpose to a waiting world!

# introduction

I sat on the edge of the sagging mattress. My clothing, now soaked with the sweat of one jolted from a deep slumber, hung on my physical frame. My body was numb, and it pressed its full weight on the box-spring, bed-frame as if my limbs and torso were crafted of molten lead.

The heart within me beat in an agitated state like a hummingbird somewhere between feeding and flight, as a swirl of thoughts—condemning, sharp, painful thoughts—punctuated the air around my head, and in a mystical, mental-spiritual transfer became darts that pierced into my inner soul.

A cry escaped from my now parched lips; the only cry that could express the depths of the agony within **"They took my baby!"**

However, lest you misunderstand, *mine was not the loss of a physical child.* I am not a woman that I should know the agonies of a miscarriage or death of an offspring that I had carried to term; I am a man.

A man nonetheless, a citizen of the Kingdom of the Beloved, who sitting on the bed's edge faced the unkind reality that his child: a vision that was conceived in his spiritual womb; that was carried through sleepless nights, tears and travail; a vision that he birthed, coddled, fed and nurtured to a place of maturity had been taken away.

A child whose conception was heralded with much promise in the Kingdom's corridors and humble awe by the one who was chosen to carry it to term, an offspring whose birth was attended with great joy by all the Kingdom citizens near the place of nativity was now removed from his care; a parent deemed no longer fit to guide the one he sired.

Had I known that like the Bible's Mary my heart would eventually be pierced by the one I bore, I might have foregone the nights of intimacy with my Beloved, ignoring His words of affection, turning my back on His wooing and purposely guarding my spiritual womb from the seeds of His vision and purpose.

Or had I attempted but not effectively blocked the seed, I eventually might have aborted the vision in the night hour when the accuser of my soul bade me so.  But, I did neither.

And once pregnant with His purpose, out of love for the Beloved, I carried the child of purpose and potential to full term, nurtured and protected him until that fateful day.

---

My child had not died that day, but my role as caregiver: of nurture, protection and direction had forever ceased.

And like parents throughout the millennia, I wondered if I had said enough, done enough or instilled enough into the child's upbringing. Had I laid a sufficient foundation that would allow my baby to thrive without my daily words of wisdom, oversight and warm touch?

I also, like the millennia's parents, knew the feeling of the emptiness of a nest, where a chick, long flown, leaves an expansive space in the home and heart; where the mementos of a thousand memories and the photos of the years now gone are all that remain of one's pride and joy.

---

Somewhere, in the emptiness of that moment on the edge of my mattress, a faint but familiar voice echoed through time, called out from Eden's garden and whispered in my ear: **"Kingdom Citizen, this is not the end of purpose or destiny for your life!"**

My heart stirred as I wiped the tears from my now moist cheeks. In the midst of shock and grief I knew, once my heart was mended, that He could again do in me and through me what He had done only a few short years before.

## the lifecycle of a vision

A vision starts out as a small seed, planted through intimacy with the Beloved into the spiritual womb of a willing vessel who wrestles through the sleepless—but prayer filled— nights, the agony of spiritual travail, and the birthing pangs of that which they were entrusted to carry to term.

In the hour of labor, the vision on the inside is pushed out and presented to the waiting world. Great Kingdom promise is   up in the initial fetal stage; in time developing into a plump little bundle of drooling, attention-demanding joy: an infantile program, ministry or outreach that has world-changing potential.

Through years of nurture and care—from the midwife who attends the birth to the nanny who prepares and administrates the long list of the vision's needs—the baby becomes a child and hopefully survives into adulthood. As it reaches maturity, the vision's potential influence grows broad and its integrity deep, while parental influence decreases as they move off the scene and commit their grown child into the care of others.

The landscape of the Kingdom is populated with the fruit of multiple healthy births: institutions, ministries, programs and outreaches that reflect His heart and have influenced the destinies of masses of humanity.

It is a Kingdom truth that Intimacy with the Beloved always leads to the planting of the seed of vision, purpose and power in the willing spiritual womb of His Bride. And, the Beloved doesn't practice birth control!  Regardless of age, gender or status, every time Divinity and Humanity meet together in intimacy, purpose is planted, destiny and dreams are developed, and world-changing concepts are conceived.

# conception

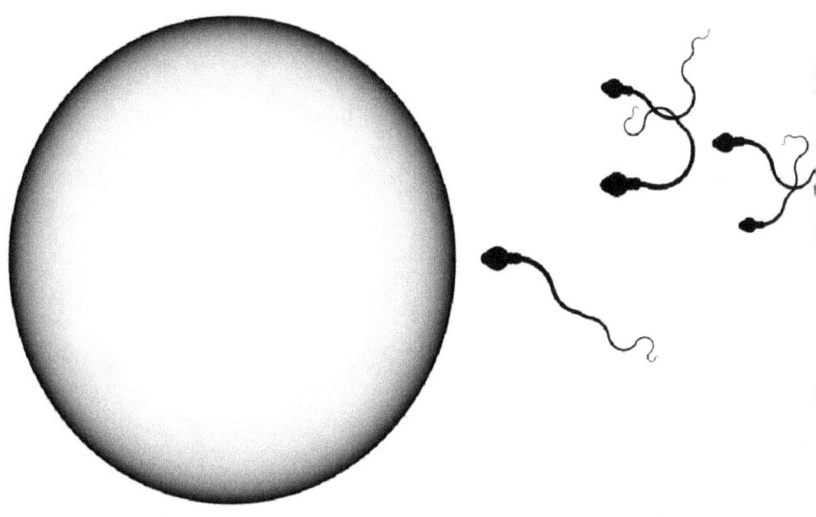

## intimacy with Him

The night air was thick with the expectancy of my Beloved's arrival. Since the moment of our first meeting, I found myself longing for none other but the nearness of His presence and His comforting, warm embrace.

I met Him first over two decades before as a confused youth, trapped in a state of soul brokenness, spiritual darkness and a tormenting mental distress—a distress accentuated by the piercing drone of a choir of ever-present demonic voices.

As I followed the bidding of the voices, and made improper choices and nurtured unholy spiritual alliances, my moral fiber began to unravel, and the ground of my being was as sand sifting through the narrow opening in an hourglass.

With each passing moment I found first a leg, then the other, my torso and upper body being squeezed, and with the weight of the pressure on my life both pressed and pulled into the void below.

I had known about Him by name, but had never really known Him. I would call myself by His name, but His presence would have been unrecognizable to my hardened heart.

I could somehow believe that He was real, because I saw the change in my peers who claimed relationship with Him: a once drugged, teen crowd whose glazed eyes and hollow faces were one day amazingly replaced with a magnetic glow.

Yet, in my limited youthful perspective my intellect reasoned that the sands of time would only sift through the hole of the hourglass for so long.

Feeling the foundation already shifting and sifting beneath my feet, I recognized that my fate was sooner or later to be sucked into what I perceived was the blackness and bleakness on the other side of this thing called life.

With a head full of voices and a heart filled with unquantifiable pain, in my distress I accepted the lie that there was not hope, nor Beloved's cross to save from the pain of life or the uncertainty of the next.

I decided that I would enter the great abyss beyond life sooner than later and end the confusion of youth. It was at that moment, walking on a tightrope poised between despair and eternity, when He first stepped in.

---

One might argue that He was there all the time, but for years He graciously waited in the side-lines of my life, storing up a mother's prayers and waiting for the moment when I would realize my miserable estate and cry out for His mercy.

He knew the split second when my foot would slip off the tightrope of time as He patiently waited to snatch me from a premature step over into eternity.

His hand caught me during a night of swaying choirs, the clapping and raising of hands among a people called by His name expressing their affection and gratitude to Him.

That night, it was as if His presence walked in the cool of the garden again, bypassed Adam and all the others and personally called me by name.

As I felt His nearness, I collapsed under the weight of the heavy chains that gripped my feet and the shackles that held my hands and heart in bondage.

He touched me in a way that night that I could never forget, so much so that if the temptation to return to unbelief ever presented itself I could never in my heart say that He wasn't real.

In the midst of a life of brokenness, hypocrisy and deception, He came to meet me in the place within and his presence forever changed my life.

It was He that night that silenced the inner demons that left screaming as my life was transferred from a dark, dank place to the Kingdom of the Beloved: a place that flooded my mind with light illuminable.

I rose from the floor of my deliverance that night, bruised, rough around the edges and terrified within; and like Paul on the Damascus road not fully comprehending what had just occurred, but touched for eternity.

The events of that night were the beginning of a long-term transformative relationship. Over the years, He came many times and initiated a process that melted away the layers of the hard and crusty exterior that had been a weak protection for my bruised and bleeding interior.

As if I was an onion, His hand pealed back each smelly, sticky piece; touching and taking only that which I could release. He became for me a salve for my heart until the bleeding subsided and the wounds dried up and scabbed over— He was my Beloved.

## the soul's retreat

It was a calm night in the early spring. The activities of the day past had ended as I retreated to the quiet of an inner room, expectantly awaiting His coming.

As I had so many times before, I desired again to experience the closeness of His embrace and the heavy press of His presence: that tangible weightiness of His Glory in the room.

In the solitude of that evening, I longed for Him once again to draw near to my side and whisper words of life in my ear, words expressing His desire and heart for me. Words infused with a hot spiritual fire that could ignite the kindling of my dry heart.

I was an addict—intimacy with him was a primary pursuit in my life.

It was a goal in whose pursuit caused me for seasons to push away from the table of food and the warmth of human companionship.

A goal in whose reward was far more satisfying than meeting a momentary biological hunger pang or the sociological gratification of a need for human contact. He had become the source of my joy.

---

There is an attitude of waiting that only a lover can understand. It is the combination of a rapid heartbeat and increased adrenaline level, a balancing the tension of keeping oneself in a patient place, quiet, calm, while every fiber of one's being sits expectantly on the edge of a metabolic chair looking for the entry of the object of one's affection.

As I patiently waited for Him that night, the perfumed scent of His presence preceded His entry and began to seep into the room, saturating the atmosphere of the moment.

Whether it was a real fragrance I did not know, but upon first breath, it brought sweetness, as honey, to my spirit, and calmness to my racing heart.

In a fitting response, I bowed reverently towards the floor. Not in the cute curtsey of one in the presence of human royalty, fulfilling the dictates of social manners; but as one in the presence of a beneficent, transcendent royalty.

Words of adoration slid down my tongue, and, like water bouncing off the pebbles in a brook, stumbled across my stammering lips, sounding less like my mother tongue and more like a heavenly cacophony as the evening progressed.

That night I reveled in the nearness of Him. And as our encounter progressed and I basked in His presence, my words suddenly stopped and I found myself sitting in silence.

It was out of necessity that my words had to cease lest they became a hindrance, for the rest of the night was His to pour out into me a transfer of grace: an imparting of His Spirit that was like fresh water to my parched soul.

It was during that night of intimacy that He planted a seed in that undefined area of my inner self: my spiritual womb.

My heart was a receptive channel, His presence was near and penetration took place somewhere in the midst of my adoration and the silence of my tongue.

The planted seed was small, but was firmly encased in a shell of potential and promise. The seed was a vision for a people-impacting program.

As my mind, lagging behind and understanding only in part the spiritual transfer that had just taken place, raced to catch-up, I took out a paper and pencil and began to sketch out the details of the vision.

I filled one side of a page of notebook paper with broad brushstrokes and the other with the finer details of a picture yet to be painted.

The vision was at the same time something internal, small and ill-defined for the moment, yet also clearly laid out on the paper.

Although I could not conceive how or when the birth would take place, and wondered why I had been chosen for such a task, I knew that a tangible transaction had taken place and the thing would become a reality in the Beloved's timing.

## a visitation

For too long we have heard a message that gives the false impression that we are the ones who bring the weight of His glory into a room through our worship.

We have mistaken that His promise to inhabit our praise (Ps 22:3) meant that somehow He was at our beckon call.

We somehow became the sole initiators of the divine-human relationship. And as the initiators, we invited His presence and power into our lives and assemblies when it suited our agenda or comfort level.

Could it be that in the midst of our worship we bypassed true intimacy with our Beloved for a relationship that we subconsciously believed we could turn off and on at will; a relationship in which He became our cosmic servant, our pacifier and a medicinal salve for whatever ailed our souls, bodies or pocketbooks.

In our ignorance, our actions demoted Him from His position of greatness, and brought Him down to a position of servitude to our place of need.

In our Kingdom assemblies, His presence was welcome during the opening prayer and three worship songs, as long as we could be finished with our program and out of the building within the hour.

Or His touch was desired and eagerly sought during trauma or duress like a bandage that stops the bleeding but is later unceremoniously discarded in the trash bin.

Somewhere in our ignorance, we have lost the sense of His sovereignty, and our place as His servants; the understanding that it was His love that sought us, continues to cry out from Calvary and scout through the trails of eternity until it finds us hiding in the crevices of time.

That in the beginning hours of creation it was His knee that bent and hands that formed our being from the dust of the earth. It was His mouth that breathed into us; like a lifeguard resuscitating a drowning man, with His own breath; the very breath of life.

---

Even in humanity's darkest hour, when in paradise we turned our backs on His command, even though we had all provision for happiness and sustenance, because we were temped to grasp divinity—it was not we who searched for Him, but He who "*walked in the cool of the day*" in the garden calling us by name.

Yet, even with the benefit of historic hindsight, we still like Eden's first couple have all hid from the presence of our Beloved because of an acute awareness that we have fallen short of His Glory.

In our modern-day enactment of the first couple's desperate fear of exposure, we have crafted the fig-leaves of human effort, mental and physical development and religion to hide the fact that we are naked.

The fig leaves keep us hidden from each other and from the One who made us.

Could it be that our worship has become a fig leaf? Somewhere in our fear of intimacy with Him, that we invoke His presence only within the level of our comfort, and only as long as we are near the psycho-spiritual switch that can quickly be flipped to "off" when the cool of the garden is disrupted by His voice.

---

It is He who initiates intimacy with our souls. It is He who invites us to disrobe the frail garments that we craft to hide our brokenness.

And, should we be unable or unwilling to disrobe, the winds of His Spirit gently blow through our lives and leaves, with the combination of the gusts of a strong storm, mingled with a soft touch, defoliating the barriers that keep us from Him.

**There is an hour of His visitation where it is not us initiating the praise, or pressing in to seek Him, but He is the initiator and we the passive recipients of His visit.**

## now I lay me down

The Divine Lover cannot love if the object of His affection does not relinquish control. When He seeks for us and calls us by name, we cannot run and hide from His presence.

Instead, we must come to the place where we stop our running, cease the noise and scurry of activity, and sit receptively before Him; fig leaves removed, naked before our

God, allowing Him to pour His love into our hearts.

How can a human lover ravish the tokens of his affection on his beloved if she will not lay in his presence, relax and entrust her body and soul to his caress? How can she receive if she is not in a receptive posture before him?

How can the divine interplay between the Son and His bride take place if the bride refuses to let Him take the lead, and spends her waking hour scurrying to and fro in endless ministry activity?

When He beckons us we must be the ones to respond to His call: slowing down, relinquishing our control, placing ourselves in an obvious receptive mode—waiting for Him.

———————————————

Jesus' friend Mary sat at His feet, enjoying his presence and when her sister Martha, scurrying around in acts of service, remonstrated, He said, "*Mary has chosen what is better, and it will not be taken away from her*" (Luke 10:42; NIV).

Did Jesus intend to communicate to us that Martha's service was unappreciated—or that service in general is not useful—I think not!

He was simply making the point that when the Son of Man enters your house and comes to sup at your table, it is a special event that should cause you to pull aside from the routine of daily life, including even sacrificial acts of service, to sit at his feet.

When Mary the prostitute broke her costly alabaster box of ointment and anointed Jesus' feet with the oil, wiping it with her hair, and the disciple in charge of financial matters noted that the money from the ointment could have been used to feed the poor; Jesus replied that "*the poor you will always have with you*" (Matt. 26:11; NIV).

Was Jesus intending to belittle the ministry of compassion and service to the poor—definitely no!

The point was that in the hour of His visitation, we must focus our hearts, minds and bodies on responding to His special presence in our midst; meeting His needs as it were, instead of the needs that are always around us.

————————————————————————

Giving up control is not sliding into a passive fatalistic state where the being becomes devoid of thought or passion.

Giving up control is simple surrender to the desire of the Beloved; that in the midst of thought and passion we give up our right to know what is coming next to allow Him the sole authority to shape and direct what He does in us, with us and through us.

Contrary to passivity, the loss of control means that He is allowed to initiate in us that which is pleasing to Him. Our role is to respond to His word and wooing with the mixture of joy and awe that should naturally accompany His presence.

To the Beloved a passive response to His embrace is an unfulfilling response. What lover wants to make love to a lifeless, unresponsive mate, whose presence in the act of intimacy is out of duty instead of true delight?

The Beloved desires and delights when a mixture of submission and passion is our response to His wooing call; that we would become active participants in the love relationship; His pleasure stirred when our passion is ignited by His presence.

## a bed of trust

Allowing the Beloved to ravish you with the tokens of His affection is only possible in a bed of trust: a bed that is made through years of experiencing His presence and provision.

A trust that if you become truly transparent and allow Him close to you that He will not condemn you or cast you off for what He sees in your life.

A trust that if you are broken like the proverbial reed, that "*a bruised reed He will not break!*" (Matt. 12:20; NIV).

The enemy of trust is the fear of loosing control. Fear of not being able to set the agenda and manipulate the outcomes for the relationship will cause one's heart to remain closed to His presence, and life hidden from His healing touch and warm embrace.

Refusing to relinquish the role of initiator in the relationship due to insecurity will stifle the ability to receive all that He desires to lavish upon one.

In the Bible, it was the Psalmist's Beloved that traversed the crags, leaped on the mountains and skipped on the hills searching for the object of His longing.

The Beloved patiently seeks for us in the same way. It is in His visitation in the garden and in our lives, and our hearts response to his wooing that the divine/human love relationship is played.

---

A bed that is not cushioned with trust will either result in a night of sweaty rumbling that lacks of intimacy or a night of frigidity.

The rumbling may produce a child but will lack the bond of love and commitment needed to sustain the relationship long term, with the birth-parent eventually drifting far from the Beloved's presence, and in a sort of divine/human divorce separating from the Father of the child they carry.

The frigid bed is covered with questions of the Beloved's motives. It produces a romance that is cursed with suspicion over the Beloved's every action and a resultant closed heart that refuses to fully trust His presence and touch.

Should He gently touch the brow of His intended, and push back the loose strands of hair to see their eyes, they quickly turn their head to avoid His piercing stare.

There is no possibility for true affection or impregnation because the object of the Beloved's attention is tightly closed up from His presence.

To expose the heart of the intended, the Beloved has been known to leave the room and presence of the object of His affection momentarily.

For the Kingdom Citizen whose bed is made with trust, they miss the nearness of His touch, but never doubt His love or care.

Should there be an apparent delay in His return to the room, they wait calm, still and expectantly for His return, knowing that although he may not feel near, He is always within range should they call out His name.

They ultimately understand that His plan and presence is worth the wait.

For those not resting in a bed of trust, when the Beloved appears to leave the room, the reaction is similar to a person put on extended hold on the telephone.

Although the recorded message promises that the call will soon be answered, even to the estimate of minutes until the promise is fulfilled, the caller responds with irritation, impatience and anger, eventually turning into despair and unbelief that the call will ever be answered.

Without trust, the Beloved's delays ultimately reveal the gulf in a relationship that should be close, and the lack of the trust and intimacy needed for impregnation to occur.

# the open womb

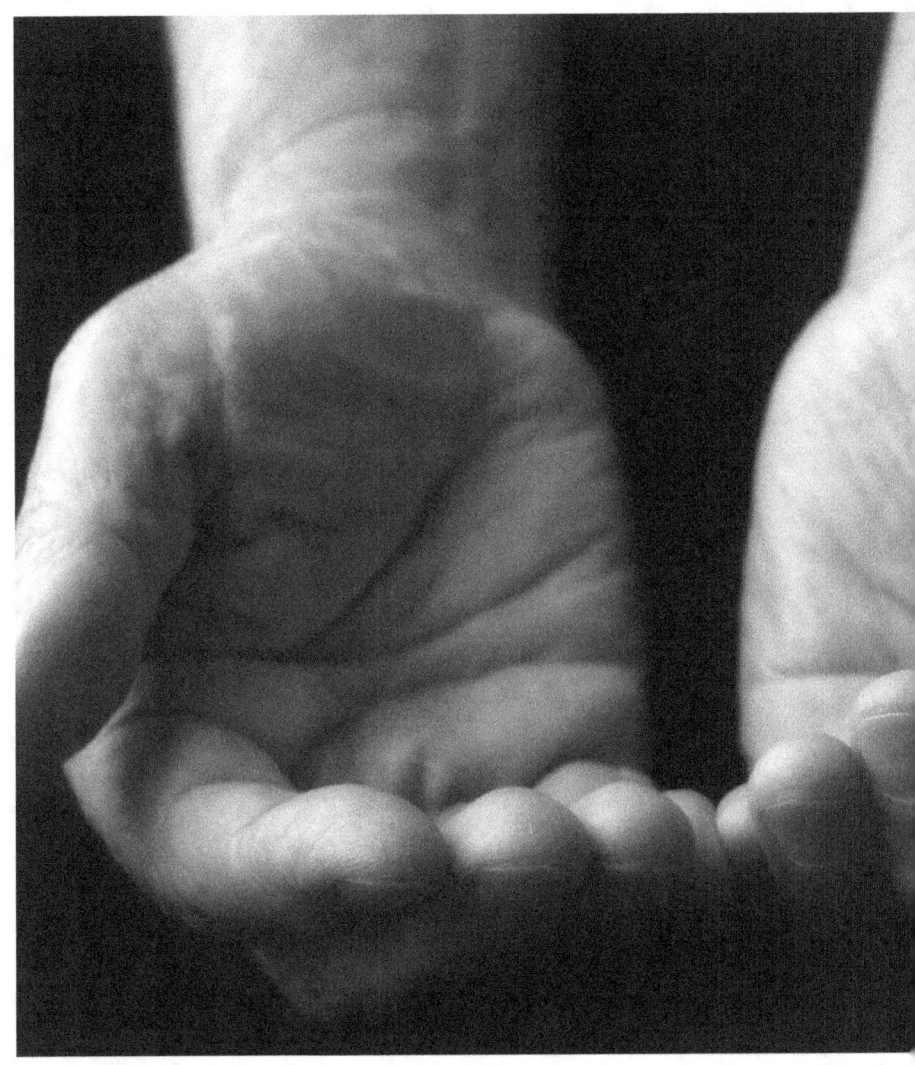

# be it unto me

*"And Mary said, Behold, the handmaid of the Lord; be it unto me according to thy word"* (Luke 1:38; NASV).

In the annals of the Kingdom, one stands above all others as the greatest historical example of a receptive vessel: Mary the mother of Jesus.

A virgin betrothed to her fiancé, Joseph, she was visited by an angel of the Lord who at once told her that she was highly favored and the Lord was with her (Luke 1:28, 30; NASV).

Following the message of divine favor and encouragement, the heavenly visitor began to speak about Mary conceiving in her womb; and of her son spoke a litany of greatness that he would be the Son of the Most High, receive the throne of his father David, reign over the house of Jacob for ever and rule over a Kingdom that would have no end.

To this litany Mary's response was an innocent, if not naive: *"how shall this be, seeing I know not a man."* (Luke 1:34; NASV).

When the angel replied that the Holy Spirit would come upon her, and the power of the most high God would overshadow her: *"wherefore the holy thing that is begotten shall be called the son of God"* (Luke 1:35; NASV); Mary replied with her famous words: *"be it unto me according to thy word!"*

When met with the unsettling oracle of a radiant heavenly creature, Mary saw her lack: she had never been intimate with a man, and she knew that babies only came through intimate relations with the opposite sex.

When instructed that the Holy Spirit of the most high God would come over her—and the child would be the child of promise that the sages had foretold, and the ages had awaited; her response became a role model for generations of chosen vessels.

*"Be it unto me according to thy word"* is the honest reply of one who would be the object of the Beloved's

affection, spreading her garments on the bed of trust, allowing Him to have His way with her until the seed of vision was planted deep in the gestating place; where the holy thing found its bed of planting.

"*Be it unto me*" is the response of one not impressed by the fact that they have never been pregnant or birthed before.

It is, in essence, the only reply suitable to the Divine Lover, who saw a purity and willingness of heart in Mary, as He does in us when He visits us with a word, or promise of purpose and destiny.

———————————————

In the hour of our visitation, we may wonder at the words of the message, and question the status of our ability to conceive; but it is when the Beloved Himself validates the call to conception with the promise of His overshadowing our human limitations that our response should parallel Mary's willingness.

Having an open spiritual womb means the interior place in our being will become home for and nurture something that will grow bigger than, and beyond our greatest expectations and human limitations.

As a type of surrogate parent, we get the privilege of being a vessel to carry another's vision, and the other just happens to be the Beloved.

An open spiritual womb means that the tender, nutritiously lined place that is the fountainhead of personal prayer, spiritual ministry and Kingdom fruit will welcome one that will attach itself in dependence and over the months draw from its lifeline of intercession and spiritual power as it develops and grows.

And from that inner tender place, the protected vision will be able to form from the smallest of frames until the moment when the thing has grown so huge that it is pressed against the nutritious walls until they are able to stretch no more; and feeling the constraints of its surroundings, and waiting to transition outside to its destiny, it begins to kick the boundaries of the womb of the willing vessel.

## God doesn't practice birth control

There is a spiritual truth that you will not find described in the terms I will use in the tomes of theology, or the lecture halls of sacred academia: the truth that "*God doesn't practice birth control.*"

Every incidence in the Bible when a man or woman of God had an intimate relationship with the Lord, a baby was produced.

For Mary and Hannah it was a flesh and blood baby. For Noah the baby was a big wooden ark; for Paul it was the greater part of the New Testament and the foundations of the Christian Church.

**Every time that Divinity and Humanity meet together in Intimacy; Kings and Saviors, and World Changing Organizations and Movements are Birthed!**

It is parallel to that of a human relationship. When a man and woman come together in intimate relations, the only thing that will stop the natural process of conception from eventually taking place is what we so aptly call "birth control": an apparatus whose sole purpose is to keep the aggressive sperm from finding its way to the fertile egg.

Our society is so conditioned to self-fulfillment and the abandonment to that which gives us pleasure that many have almost forgotten that the joys and release found in "intimate relations" with the opposite sex, while fostering human pleasure, serve in a grander design to promote the propagation of the human race.

It is almost as if the Divine reasoning foresaw that humanity would not naturally choose to procreate, going through the agony of pregnancy and the birthing of babies if there were not the intense pleasure associated with the act of copulation.

Despite the divine reasoning, we have creatively made it possible to have the pleasure without the resultant conception and birth.

In our relationship to Him many have taken on a self-centered view that presupposes that His highest good, aim and reason for existence is to make us happy and meet our needs.

In this world-view, worship becomes that which makes me feel good. I delight in the intimacy of His presence; desire that He would hold me close, touch me and speak His good pleasure to me—but I don't want to become pregnant or carry His babies.

To this mindset we want our relationship to Him to be forever just like it was the first time we met; when it was the two of us—me enraptured in His presence, lost to time and space because of the intensity of His love poured out in my life.

We want to eternally live in the rush of the prom-night kiss, preserving the corsage in the deep freeze until it dries to dust, keeping the photos of that one night forever etched in our mind and sealed in the plastic photo album, next to the unread Bible, on the coffee table of our heart.

But, while the memory of that one night is precious, and worthy of being remembered and testified to, it is a poor substitute for a growing relationship with the Beloved that increases in intimacy over time and leads to the eventual birthing of vision.

Certainly, pregnancy doesn't feel good and children can mess up one's step. But fostering the attitude that "All I want it to be is Jesus and me, alone, with no children!" will leave your relationship with the Beloved stuck somewhere between the memories of that one night stand and the flower dust moldering in the fridge.

## the master's desire

The Beloved wants to draw near to us, touch and heal us for one purpose: that **out of the intimacy of our relationship to Him He can impregnate us with the seed**

**of vision.**

The Bible says that *"where there is no vision, the people perish"* (Proverbs 29:18; KJV). The Kingdom and Beloved's purposes are stalled when there is no vision. Our individual lives become unfulfilled and aimless when we are not motivated by a vision.

It is Kingdom vision planted in our spiritual womb, carried through agonizing nights and days of discomfort, pushed into reality through our spiritual birth canal that is the Beloved's desire.

He chooses to use us for His purposes, and draws us into His presence—so that out of intimacy will be birthed something so precious that our sphere of influence, small or gargantuan, will be changed for eternity. **In the spirit, God never practices birth control!**

⊢―――――――――――――――――⊣

The Beloved is not practicing birth control, but are we? In natural human relations, we have the option of blocking the sperm from the seed—enjoying the pleasure without the resultant conception—even so, it is in the spiritual.

We can enjoy the intimacy of the time spent with the Beloved, yet refuse to become impregnated with the seed of His purpose for our lives.

### Spiritual birth control takes two forms: the Diaphragm of Disobedience or the Prophylactic of Pride.

We can draw near to Him but don the diaphragm of disobedience to keep His seed from ever reaching or taking hold of anything in our spiritual womb.

Disobedience blocks the seed of vision from our inner self. We disobey when we ignore or reject that which He attempts to reveal to us in our times of intimacy; acting like we didn't hear His voice, or, shutting off our conscience in a self-deceiving denial.

A truth about the Beloved's character is that He is not a forceful lover. He will never abuse us by controlling or manipulating us to obey; nor will He force the seed past the barriers that we have erected in our lives.

The Beloved will never rape us in an attempt to promote His Kingdom agenda and sovereign plan for humanity.

The Chronicler said that His eyes "*run to and fro throughout the whole earth, to show Himself strong on behalf of those whose heart is loyal to Him*" (2 Chron 16:9; NKJV).

He will woo us, draw near to us, call and shower blessings, and pour oil and wine into our souls; but if we continually refuse Him, His eyes eventually will look for and find another.

No, He will not abandon us to the nether regions for eternity, but He will leave us to our prom-night memories. Leaving us sitting jaded, on a dated avocado-green, plastic-covered sofa, in our comfort zone—a small mental living room of our own making—where we repeatedly replay the video tape of that one night, and occasionally wonder what it might have been had we consummated the relationship without the diaphragm.

---

For some the birth control of choice is more insidious: we protect ourselves from the impregnation of vision with the prophylactic of pride.

The biblical definition of pride is that we think of ourselves more highly than we should (Rom 12:3).

Pride is self-intoxication, were the ego is so enraptured and impressed by itself and its accomplishments that it staggers and swaggers, drunk to and by itself—the focus being totally on self!

The prophylactic of pride is so insidious because it is the reverse of the swagger and stagger pride of the inflated ego. It is the pride that thinks of ourselves not more highly, but more lowly than we should.

It is a mindset that appears self-effacing and humble,

as the one donning the prophylactic is constantly downplaying their contribution, abilities and purpose.

When the Beloved comes to that one with vision and purpose, they will shrink back because they are so bound with a sense of inferiority and worthlessness that they genuinely do not believe that they are worthy of anything nearing or appearing like a grand purpose; and they question why He, the great and mighty One, would choose to use lowly and miserable them.

That which stops the seed is not the acknowledgement that there is little to nothing in us that can fulfill the purposes of God (John 15:5), but it is the refusing to acknowledge that if He is the one planting the seed, and, if He chose to come to us, He must have seen something in us that He wanted and could use.

Our role is that of passive womb, receiving and faithfully carrying that which He plants. When the prophylactic of pride is on, the focus even in the midst of self-effacement is still 'self'!

---

For too many in the Kingdom, they carry the pain of disappointment or hurt that is so great that they avoid His presence all-together.

Knowing that intimacy produces children, they avoid Him at all costs; His messages go unanswered on the machine, His messengers and the place of their meeting are not only ignored but also avoided.

They are the ones who once entered into His presence with abandon, experiencing all the joys of intimacy with the Beloved. They are the ones who gladly opened their hearts, minds and wombs to all the vision and potential that He could pour in.

They laid economic and educational pursuits down to become pregnant with His purpose, and gladly bore the pressure, agony and warfare to birth His babies.

But somewhere along the line the baby was killed, the

vision shattered, the child ripped to shreds by wolves in the Kingdom: people called by His name but not wed to His heart or purposes.

This one sadly practices the most successful form of birth control in any of the kingdoms of man or the Beloved: abstinence.

Abstaining from all relations with the Beloved; going out of their way to avoid His presence; pulling out and re-donning the primal fig leaves and running from the sound of His voice in the garden of their lives.

Avoiding all the gatherings and trappings of Kingdom life, they pull away from Him, because sadly those who purported to be from Him and of Him were the cause of the death of the one they bore.


## a heart's cry

The priest had not seen such a drunken woman in all the days of his ecclesiastical duties; an obviously frustrated being who rocked and beat the floor with an intensity that caused the dust on the stones to fill the air.

Moving closer to the corner of the temple where she prayed, he observed that her muscles were tensed as one in extreme agony, and her lips moved but no words came out of her mouth.

This woman who lay prostrate on the altar was the Bible's Hannah. One of two wives of a man called Elkanah; she was barren while her peer wife, Peninnah, had a full and fruitful womb.

Hannah was a frustrated woman. Every year when Elkanah, his wives and children went to the temple to worship, Hannah's heart broke because her womb was barren and her peer's fruitful.

She longed to have the disgrace of her dead, empty womb wiped away with the fruitfulness that came from being in the family way!

Hannah's husband loved his first wife despite her

barrenness. He showered the tokens of his affection on her attempting to fill the void in her life caused by no babies she could call her own.

But, even with his verbal and physical affection, Hannah still felt a void of purpose in her life that could be met by no man, even her mate.

She knew that her dead womb was created for fruitfulness, and that God alone could restore life to a dead place.

As she bore the frustration of her barrenness, she pressed into God in the place of prayer until we find her as this chapter opened in an agonizing moment of travail before God where her bitterness of soul left her with no words, and her lips stammered as a woman inebriated.

It was in that moment that her desperate heart cried out from the depths of her being that God remembered her, opened her womb, and granted to her pregnancy and the birth of the prophet Samuel.

---

For many called to birth vision there is the inevitable season of frustration experienced before conception. It is frustration, responded to by prayer that propels one toward conception.

Like us, Hannah may never have moved to a place of crying out to God had it not been for the provocation of her peer wife, who vexed her sorely.

She had her husband's loyalty and affection, and his acceptance of the fact that she could never bare him an offspring; he loved her despite her barrenness.

Hannah could have accepted her dead womb and lived a comfortable life as her husband's first wife, receiving his unconditional love, and provision of food, shelter and raiment were it not for her provocation.

**Many in the Kingdom have accepted barrenness wrapped in a sterile and sympathetic comfort that would go unchecked except for the occasional spiritual Peninnah, sent to challenge the calm and stir up the depths of disquiet.**

The calm acceptance of barrenness and deadness is disrupted as we begin to feel the provocation of our Peninnah who over time ups the ante to a place set above our limitations and causes us to reevaluate what we thought the Beloved could or could not do in our lives.

While we formerly were content with our little house, and meals and the affection of our human companions, we begin to see that we are missing that which will bring the deepest satisfaction: the birthing of vision.

In the hour of provocation, the vexation on the outside of our lives is met with pressure on the inside and a mental and emotional storm that attempts to erode the stability of our minds and hearts.

The provoking storm is sent to press us into a deeper place of prayer.

It is a truth experienced by many in the Kingdom that, when we are at ease in Zion, we will not want to carry and birth Zion's children; when provoked from outside and in with the fact that our ease is not the Kingdom's best, we will cry out for vision to be planted in our womb.

$$\longmapsto\joinrel\joinrel\joinrel\joinrel\joinrel\joinrel\joinrel\joinrel\joinrel\joinrel\joinrel\joinrel\joinrel\joinrel\joinrel\longleftarrow$$

Unfortunately many, especially men, never make it past the place of frustration to the birthing room.

Without much thought or understanding as to what we are experiencing, we instinctively recoil from the slightest hint of the pain that will be involved in birthing the baby the Beloved wants to plant within.

Instead of leaning in and pressing through what is intended to propel us toward destiny, we instead pull back from the frustration in our hour of provocation, and retreat to mind numbing or body stimulating activities.

As men, we can attempt to sympathize with a woman's burden during pregnancy and her travail and agony in the physical birthing process, but we can never truly relate to or understand it.

A woman in labor bears a level of agony that no man, even under the greatest duress, could ever comprehend.

There is nothing in the male experience that even comes close to the heavy load that grows inside and the labor that physically rests upon an expectant mother.

In the realm of spiritual work, the women of the Kingdom often seem to have an innate capacity to enter in and wrestle with the confusion, tension, enemy attack, and excruciating pain that goes with giving birth to what God plants.

For the male, he will have to move beyond the discomfort of carrying a big thing in his belly, refuse to pull back into the numbing/stimulating activities and learn to press into the spiritual birthing process.

For the Kingdom son or daughter, seasons of frustration must be met with a pressing in to the Beloved's presence instead of a pulling back; a leaning into instead of a fleeing.

The frustration will often be misunderstood, as all the components of life that make for happiness: the affection of the husband despite the barren womb, as it were, will be in place.

But the dis-ease even in the midst of favor can be a signal that there is more that the Beloved has for you; that living contently with all the trappings of apparent divine favor yet accepting a barren womb is a life unlived.

———————————————————

Hannah pouring out her heart in frustration before the Lord produced not only a first-fruits of her womb: a son who she dedicated totally to the Lord—she was blessed with many more small lives that graced her home and brought fulfillment to her once provoked life.

In reward for her willingness to give up her first son, the Bible records that "*the Lord was gracious to Hannah; she conceived and gave birth to three sons and two daughters...*" (1 Sam 2:21; NIV).

## stripping of reliance on the flesh

The truly great children of vision are not born into the Kingdom because of human prowess, cleverness or beauty.

Although there are many in our time that birth babies based on the beauty and impressiveness of their own flesh— the ability to package, market and dress the frame of the ordinary child so that they appear to be world-transforming— those that are the truly great in the Kingdom are born where the human parent has no reliance or confidence in their flesh.

The Beloved enjoys choosing the one who lives socially, educationally and economically on the proverbial "wrong side of the tracks". This is the one who initially elicits no turned heads when seen promenading down the boulevards of the Kingdom.

They are the one, who like King David, came from the wrong family, and were the least likely to be chosen from within that family. They are the one of whom is said: "*can any good thing come out of Nazareth?*" (John 1:46).

No, the one He chooses does not have place for their flesh to boast. Their greatness comes from Him alone, a fact which they know all too well, and the result in that the credit of their exploits and success return back to Him alone.

Others who see the fruit of their spiritual loins in the vision they birth will not hesitate to acknowledge the Beloved in the works of this one's hands, because of intimately knowing the lack and weakness of the vessel.

There is a process that the Beloved takes all potential vision-carriers through; a process whose end result is that

the carrier will echo the confession of the apostle that
"...*in my flesh, dwelleth no good thing...*" (Rom 7:18).

The process may take mere months or excruciatingly
stretch out over a life-time.

The key factor determining the length of the process is
the willingness of the potential vision-carrier to lay down all
rights to self-preservation. The sooner one reaches the futility
of living life on their terms, dies to self-effort—the sooner the
process is complete.

But should one refuse to give up control, it may mean
decades of life on the back-side of the desert herding sheep
because one slew the Egyptian in their life, seeking to deliver
their people by their own power and prowess, in a time-frame
not ordained.

The process is well planned and choreographed. It is
as if one matriculates into the School of the Beloved, and
finds that they are enrolled in classes that they never signed
up for and would have avoided had they known the painfulness
of the tests.

Tests of rejection, misunderstanding, suffering and
persecution; and by far the hardest: feeling like a "nobody",
apparently going nowhere—left on the back shelf of the
Kingdom pantry, overlooked when others around are called
forward and employed in active and apparently fruitful service.

For the one submitted to Kingdom purposes, the desired
outcome of the School of the Beloved is that the tests will
produce a complete emptying of self, and an awareness that
there is no talent, gift, skill or power in one's self that will ever
be able to promote, progress or push into the public eye the
one who has been so dealt with.

After graduation from the divine program, instead of
coming to the Beloved with full hands: opinions, an agenda,
demands—this one acknowledges and lifts up empty hands
and looks to the Beloved to fill them with good things.

When one's womb is full of personal creativity, great cleverness of thought and shrewdness of activity; when one believes that they are sufficient in and of themselves to produce Kingdom fruit, there is no room for the Beloved to plant seed.

It is the one who has refused to submit and sit still until the completion of each of the tests in the Divine school, who is impressed with and relies on their accomplishments and self-sufficiency that will need to be dealt with until they see the futility of their ways except that the Beloved intervene.

**It is only when we get to the place of recognizing the emptiness of our womb—and our total inability to produce anything of ultimate value aside from His penetrating touch—that we assume the position of a Hannah and cry out with stammering lips for divinity to stoop to the vacancy of a barren womb and impregnate us for His purposes.**

It is the one who comes with empty hands, a vacant and dead womb, with no hope in themselves of conceiving who attracts the attention of the Giver of Life.

For the one who through ignorance, impatience or arrogance has not been so dealt with by the Beloved, they will forever be full of self and should they bring forth children, they will unfortunately lack the pure lifeblood of the Kingdom and the DNA of the Beloved's character.

# carrying the baby

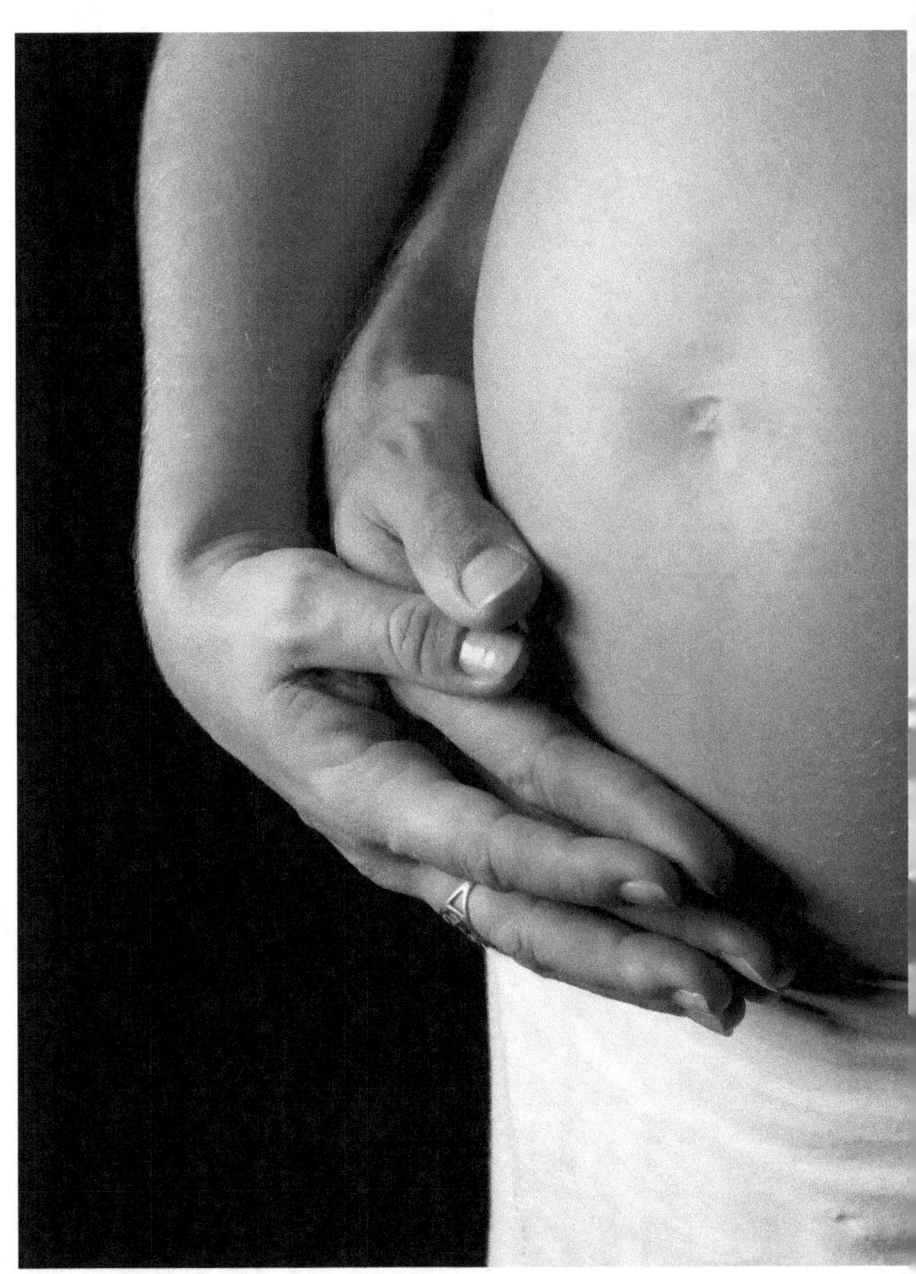

## the morning after

Without the aid of the alarm, I found myself wide awake, light streaming through the slats on the window blind, casting their streaks over the furnishings, floors and walls of my small room.

I reached over and turned off the alarm button on the clock, pushed back the covers on my bed, sat up and put my feet over the side into the slippers waiting on the floor.

Before starting my morning routine I momentarily paused on the edge of my bed, contemplating that there was something particularly fresh about the air that morning.

In fact, the whole of that day's activities were met with "freshness". My normal early-in-the-day sluggishness was over-shadowed by a burst of energy and deep joy.

You see, it was the morning after my season of intimacy with the Beloved and my heart was warmed as I reflected on the night before, and basked in His love and affirmation made so real to me.

Little did I know what was to come, but I did know this: that I was forever changed as I had been impregnated with the seed of vision in my spiritual womb.

---

As I went through my daily routine I was initially oblivious to the fact that I exhibited all the characteristics that are signature to one who is pregnant: a giddy, giggly, almost ever so slightly drunken state complete with the flush of the cheeks: a glow that attracted more attention than I wanted.

"What happened to you?" said one fellow Kingdom citizen, "You look so good, have you been working out?" said another, all sensing something had changed in me but not astute enough to understand the inner transformation that was the source of the outer transfiguration.

The freshness of the night of intimacy and the deep pleasure over the treasure that I now carried lingered for days, ever close to my thoughts and even while subsiding in intensity, still seen in the Cheshire cat grin and glassy stare that accompanied my conversations with others; that is until the day I awoke to the feeling that a three-ring circus had invaded my inner space.

--------------------------------

Little did I then understand that Kingdom pregnancy is always soon attended by a type of morning sickness: a spiritual hormonal imbalance that upsets the normal equilibrium and appears to take complete control of the physiology and psychology of the birth parent.

From a state of giddy joy I was overnight thrust into a place where my emotions took on a life of their own, ranging from a hormonal high to a place of scraping the depths and redefining the meaning of low.

Something was taking place in the realm of the spirit that I didn't understand and I really didn't appreciate.

I woke up one day to find that my clothes: the armor of God didn't fit the same as it used to.

It somehow took me longer to pray before I had the sense of receiving an answer.

Entering into worship was a task and the warfare in my mind and spirit felt intense.

My feet were bloated, and putting on the shoes of the gospel of peace, and sharing about the Beloved, took more energy and concentration; the shield of faith and the sword of the spirit were heavier and where I once wielded them with ease, I now had to focus all my energies on the task.

I despised what I was experiencing. I felt spiritually bloated and struggled to keep my emotions from busting the belt of truth that by now dug into my gut.

I don't know if I naively thought the giddy joy and afterglow of intimacy would be the prevailing experience from conception all the way to the birth of the vision—or, if I had just never really thought about the changes that attended the process of carrying vision.

But here I was feeling spiritually fat and frumpy, and wondering how my once sharp spiritual edge had apparently become so dull so quick.

The elation over being chosen to carry the Beloved's vision contrasted with the confusing emotional roller coaster of spiritual morning sickness eventually motivated me to find out if I was simply crazy or experiencing a state common to Kingdom wayfarers throughout the ages.

I eagerly hunted down, purchased and devoured any resource I could find that addressed the aspects of vision, prayer, intercession, warfare and birth.

It was here that I began to compare notes with other Kingdom citizens to find out what they experienced in the days and months that led up to the birth of their vision.

Not only did I find that I wasn't crazy, but in fact discovered the process and principles that the Beloved had established long ago, and had been understood and experienced by His citizens throughout the ages.

Through my questions and study I uncovered three distinct needs for the carrier of vision: one, the need for a proper diet during pregnancy; two, the need to control outside influences while one is nurturing their precious cargo; and, three, the need to nurture the vision behind closed lips.


## proper diet

While the vision is growing inside, a proper spiritual diet is important so it can develop in strength and health.

The small vision is attached by the chords of prayer to the spiritual womb of the birth parent. It is from that inner place where all life-giving nutrition is transferred to the developing child. It is also in that protected place that the child's early identity is formed.

For the child to enter the world in strength the parent must also be strong, consuming a diet that feeds their faith through Word and worship.

For the sake of the child, the diet should include words of encouragement of what the vision will become; its future and the influence that is destined for it on the other side of the womb.

The Beloved planted the seed of vision for a specific purpose and time, and although not all of the details may be known, the parent can be certain that every child of the Beloved has great promise and limitless potential because of its Father.

Promises of the Beloved's blessing and favor should be mixed with praise from the parent. Are there words of gratitude for being chosen for such a purpose? Is there a sense of awe and wonder at being a vision-carrier?

The child is and will be blessed, but the parent is also blessed. Even on the days when the vision seems heavy and the soul weary, the knowledge of who the Father of the vision is should be enough to draw out words of gratitude.

Doubt and pessimism from the parent are to be avoided at all cost. If the parent is not sure of the destiny of the child, they should only speak what they know and add to their speech as they add to their understanding.

If the parent never gains full understanding before the day of the birth, then simply thank the Beloved that He knows the framework and purpose of the vision within and will make it plain in time.

---

Encouragement, words of faith and prayer have the affect of expanding the inner place of the parent, which gives the developing child the space needed to grow and develop.

It is almost as if the spiritual womb is like the tent of the biblical Jabez whose tent posts can be expanded, chords pulled back and pegs strengthened to allow room for a greater blessing to be outpoured within its newly defined boarder.

The result of an expanded internal tent is that the greatness of the vision will not be stifled by the limitations of the parent.

With plenty of room to develop, the vision should eventually come forth with all its small parts in place ready for the challenges in the world.

The spiritual expansion of the parent combined with properly informing the baby of the nature of the purpose for its existence, and the potential and possibilities that await it; will make for a healthy child.

## controlled outside influences

Parallel to a proper diet was the controlling of outside influences.

Early on in the process of carrying the vision I discovered that my energy and strength were limited as I was praying for two, my own needs and that of the current development and future potential of the growing child within.

I had to take care that my limited energy was not irresponsibly dissipated into activities and relationships that were not directly focused on my vision. For the one pregnant with vision, energy misdirected is energy lost.

As a birth parent there was no more room for foolishness, coarseness, and wasting time in empty pursuits. No time for sitting around with other citizens just shooting the breeze, no room for gossip and empty talk, no place for complaining and grumbling over trivialities.

In the pregnant state, the sense of discernment was so acutely attuned to sounds, smells and emotional fluctuations that I quickly recognized that which upset my peace and disturbed my ability to focus on the child.

I noticed that many once valid expressions of social interaction and uses of personal time became tools of distraction, in the hopes that I would mis-step, slip, spiritually fall into doubt and perhaps induce a miscarriage of my precious cargo.

Very quickly, I observed the danger of environmental toxins, those poisoned words that ooze from the lips of toxic individuals, and float and fly through the air waiting for a receptive place to land and infect.

Under normal circumstances, environmental toxins can be dangerous to an individual's spiritual health, but during the vulnerable season of carrying vision, such are to be avoided at all cost.

I turned a deaf ear and walked away, limiting interaction with those who spoke questions of doubt or words of lack or defeat into the atmosphere around me.

They may not have known about my vision, because I nurtured it behind my closed lips. But, somehow, the great enemy of the soul was able to recruit some with loose lips, using them to speak words that directly challenged my ability to fulfill the call of the Beloved that rested in my belly.

In pulling aside from normal social interaction and human companionship, I know I began to appear like a hermit. But, the weight of His presence and the responsibility for His child was so heavy on my spirit that I only found relief as I turned from that which dissipated energy and responded to His presence.


## a pondering heart

"*But Mary kept all these sayings, pondering them in her heart*" (Luke 2:19)

There is a silence that must attend the lips when you carry divine potential. The vision within, only in seed form, will not be understood or accepted except by a few.

You are about to give birth to something that has the potential to forever change history in the sphere of influence that you have been assigned; breaking the boxes of religious tradition and dated social mores that have been the comfortable home and confining prison of the masses.

In the biblical record, it is recorded that Mary shared the joy of her pregnancy, and the mystery of whose child she bore only with those in her inner circle: Elizabeth and

Joseph—her confidents.

And of the two only Elizabeth fully grasped and believed the weighty story she told; while Joseph, in disbelief and shame was ready to send her away for the scandal that was wrapped up in her claims.

Forget the astounding claim that an unknown, young Hebrew girl believed that she, out of all the women who sprang from Eve's womb, was chosen to carry the savior of the world, the promised and prophesied hope of generations, in her belly.

The outrageous claim aside, Joseph was at first stuck on the fact that this unmarried, young woman who was to be his wife, who should have reserved her virginity for him alone—purported to be pregnant, and that not by him.

Were it not for the intervention of an angel in the night hour, convincing Joseph of the validity of Mary's claims to being the bearer of the Son of God; the seed that clung to the walls of Mary's inner space could have been early on aborted, or the seed carrier, the chosen vessel of the Lord, pushed socially and economically to the fringes of society forever labeled as a harlot.

After receiving her assignment, Mary pondered. She didn't rent a storefront meeting hall; get business cards; or register for her personal ministry web site.

Had Mary early on, before the fullness of time, before the actors on the stage of human and cosmic history had given her the cue for her to open her mouth, broadcast the news of that which was implanted in her womb, no one would have believed her.

Women throughout the ages had secretly wondered, fantasizing if perhaps the fruit in their womb would be the seed spoken of at the dawn of creation that would ultimately rise up and destroy the vile serpent's sting.

Out of all the women from all the generations past, who was Mary in the eyes of men to even claim to be the handmaiden of the Lord?

True vision in one's womb creates not a wild, unfettered glee but an inner celebration mixed with a holy somberness.

It was in Luke 1:46-50 that Mary said in response to her pregnancy: "*My soul doth magnify the Lord, And my spirit hath rejoiced in God my Saviour. For he hath looked upon the low estate of his handmaid: For behold, from henceforth all generations shall call me blessed. For he that is mighty hath done to me great things; And holy is his name...*"

Had Mary not pondered the seed she bore, instead choosing to publicly broadcast the news of who she was carrying—inserting her joyful announcement into a myriad of conversations at the market and the well—the enemies of God in the celestial and terrestrial realms would have lined up to devour or cause to abort the promise of God.

Mary's lips, if loose, could have led to the abortion of what she carried!

When the womb is full of gestating vision and divine potential, a calmness of spirit is necessary, as all one's energies are needed to focus on the load one carries. As in natural birth, the body will out of necessity point all its forces of nutrition, sustenance and strength to protect and grow the child.

The Bible is silent on what Mary dealt with during pregnancy. Can you imagine the normal hormonal, emotional and physical changes of pregnancy with the added knowledge that Satan, not just the minor emissaries of darkness but the ambassador of darkness himself, was waiting in the wings to encourage and help Mary miscarry or abort the seed of God?

True vision will germinate and grow in depth and influence when nurtured in a pondering heart. Lips that speak before their time are like the pudgy little fingers of a Kindergarten school child digging up her recently planted kidney bean to see if it has sprouted, and conversely risk damaging the potential of that seed from ever taking root.

It's in the warm, dark, nurturing womb of silence where the seed of vision is protected until the hour of birth. True, mature vision, while perhaps shared with a couple trusted supporters or mentors, will otherwise be attended with virtual silence until the appointed hour of travail.

When Elizabeth conceived, the Bible says that she "*hid herself five months...*" (Luke 1:24).

Both Mary and Elizabeth had a humility of spirit that rejoiced in the favor of God in the conceptions in their wombs: Mary a virgin and Elizabeth an old woman with a dried up womb; a woman whose husband referred to as "*well stricken in years*" (Luke 1:18).

Contrast the meekness and faith exhibited in Mary's pondering and Elizabeth's hiding with Zacharias, who did not believe the angel's message that he would have a son, and was told by the angel: "*behold, thou shalt be silent and not able to speak, until the day that these things shall come to pass, because thou believedst not my words, which shall be fulfilled in their season*" (Luke 1:20).

The purpose of God taking place in the gestating wombs of Mary and Elizabeth was too weighty to risk the aborting of the plan. God Himself silenced the mouth of disbelieving Zacharias since he did not already possess the heart of Mary to ponder or Elizabeth to hide.

**The truth here is that you can essentially talk away your baby!** While the vision is in its most vulnerable embryonic stages of development, the biblical multitude of counselors that is so often beneficial can bring confusion, doubt and fear when sought for advice on vision in a fetal state.

You can talk too much and unleash a flood of doubt and fear: the fruit of the words of perhaps well-meaning, but not discerning companions.

Who has not experienced the cynicism, criticism and sarcasm of friends or family who question how you could ever think that YOU were going to do or be what you felt in your gut.

They who know you best can sometimes hinder you most, if they limit your potential to what they know and have seen instead of the limitless potential that is resident in the seed of a vision from God.

# birthing the baby

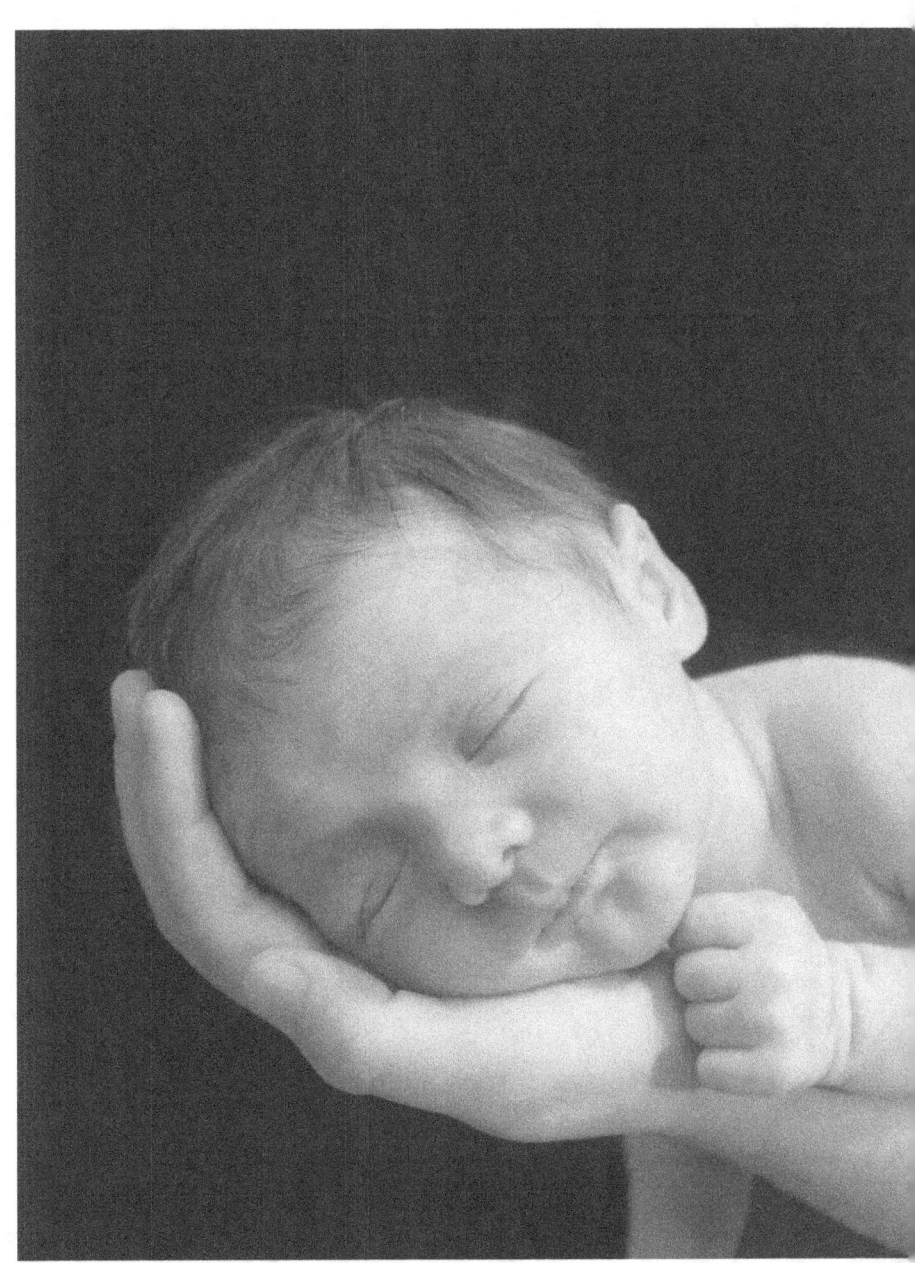

## the labor process—long nights and warfare

This night was not the first I found myself wide awake at three a.m. For a number of weeks I had not slept through the night.

It didn't matter that I retired at ten p.m. or one a.m., like the finely tuned clock on the wall in the front hallway, chiming the hour of my restlessness, I found myself propelled from the depths of sleep to a state of immediate alertness at approximately three.

The first few nights I fought this apparent interruption to my rest, quoting the Scripture that "*He gives His beloved sleep*" (Ps 127:2; NKJV); annoyed by the thought that I was wide awake and had to rise for work in a few short hours.

As I tossed and turned in my bed, I fluffed the pillows, adjusted the number of pillows, putting a fat one and a thin one together to create a proper height to rest my head; changing position on the bed, or eventually in utter disgust and frustration moving to the living room sofa.

For the initial days following the nights of unrest I analyzed my habits: from being sure I hadn't eaten too late or too much the night before; to adjusting the air temperature and thickness of blankets on the bed, all in an attempt to make sure that I was able to sleep through the night.

But, unfortunately, my travail was to no avail; without the aid of an alarm clock or complementary wake-up call, I was nightly awake at three.

---

Somewhere along the line, a few days into my sleepless spree, I remembered the words of an old gospel song: "Can't sleep at night, and you wonder why? Maybe God is trying to tell you something."

Simple words, yet a profound concept put to lyrics by one who understood that the Beloved will wake you up in the middle of the night if He has something to say, especially if your day hours are too packed to give Him the attention He deserves.

The revelation of the profoundness of those words was like a light-bulb turning on over my head. Even though I did not understand what was going on around me, I instinctively knew that I had no choice but to pray.

With my newfound understanding of the purposes of the Beloved for my night hours, I ceased struggling to fall back to sleep at three a.m., instead sitting up in my bed, and like Samuel the boy prophet asked the Lord to speak, that I, His servant, was listening.

As I woke and waited and listened, the communion with the Beloved became clearer and stronger each night. As we talked or He talked and I listened, sitting silently on my bed, every fiber of my being wrapped up in the transfer of life that took place.

The interactions usually only lasted for a couple hours; after which I rolled over and fell into a deep sleep; in truth only a short nap before the real alarm on my bed-side table clock rang to wake me, jolt me for a second time, for the day's activities.

As I awoke and waited before Him night after night, the weight of His presence grew. There was an increasing awareness that the thing He had planted in my belly was expanding inside and being prepared to come forth: my baby was kicking.

Equal was an understanding that the atmosphere that would surround the delivery was being prepped for the child.

Some nights I lay in silence, others I prayed with aggression; each night waiting until we had prayed through and the weight of His presence lifted.

Like the watchman on the walls of ancient Jerusalem, who were divided in watches of three hours; I was chosen to be up each night at the first watch to carry the burden in prayer for the purposes of the Kingdom.

Had I not obeyed the Beloved's prompting to prayer I could have prolonged labor, or missed the expected end: the birth of vision.

Through the long nights of prayer it is important to recognize that the spiritual warfare you will inevitably experience is not focused against you personally, and should therefore not be taken personally.

The dark enemy of your soul is terrified of the child that is within, and its potential to upset and do permanent damage to his kingdom rule in the hearts and minds of those the vision will touch.

You need to understand, in the late hour of the night, that the focus of the agony of the travail, and the heavy momentary presence and confusion in the thoughts due to the prince of the air is not on you but the child within.

The reality is that while you are not all that impressive, you are terrifying because you bare a seed of purpose whose father is Divine.

## the labor pains and travail

Labor pains are natural, inevitable and unavoidable to one who is pregnant and near delivery.

Labor cannot be ignored, turned off or postponed until a more convenient time, as it is all consuming: normal life activity stops, and niceties are pushed to the side as the body begins to take over with one all consuming goal—to get out what is on the inside.

Two factors are involved in labor and travail of vision: breathing and pushing. In the time of travail, the weight of the presence of the Beloved falls on one, bringing a pressure and heaviness that can only be lifted through engagement in prayer, and that not the well crafted prayer read from a book.

In the midst of the pressure, words alone will not lift the weight, as the burden does not shift by mental exercise or verbal articulateness, but by spiritual strength: the Holy Spirit within pressing and pushing even to the point of the deep groaning of prayer.

When understanding is not present in the time of prayer, communication will only come through groaning too deep for utterance (Rom 8:26); when one does not fully understand the dynamics of what is taking place in the atmosphere around—one cannot articulate the need of the hour in words of human understanding.

It is then that the intensity of wordless sounds from the Spirit praying through one will give voice to the cry of the human heart.

The weight will come, the response of pressing prayer, the weight will lift and the cycle will repeat itself again within days or hours.

The frequency in timing of the labor pains increases as one draws nearer the birth. Also increasing is the warfare and darkness. Increasing weight, increasing warfare and darkness, all responded to with pressing prayer; and increasing in frequency between incidents from weeks to days to hours, until the final moments of travail come upon the servant.

---

Somewhere in the midst of the evening watch, the Beloved says that the hour of delivery is near and the pressure within is met by an intensity without that seeks to stop the birthing of the vision.

To many, they wake to feel the enemy of their soul standing at the foot of the bed or whispering in their ear: "You really don't need to go through with this.  Why don't you close your womb, and stop the labor pangs. You are only making this up.  If your friends could see you they would think you are delusional.  What has God promised you?  Why would He put you through such agony? Abort, Abort, Abort!"

Questioning your sanity and God's integrity, his only purpose is to stop the birthing process; actually, have you stop the process and pull back from the labor and retreat from birthing the seed of God.

He knows he has no authority over the life-generating birthing process and knows he ultimately cannot stop God from bringing forth His will, and is terrified by that seed of promise that you have so faithfully carried to this final moment.

So, he is limited to feeding you lies and attempting to convince you that abortion is the best choice for your sleepless-night self.

Your choice is twofold: one, you can give ear to this dark prince's words and doubt what you thought the Beloved said to you, your credibility in carrying it out, or doubt the plans of the Beloved.

Or, two, you can press forward with the pushing and breathing, and let the outward attack be a motivating signal that deliverance is nigh; remembering that the level of the intensity of the darkness pressuring you to abort is parallel to the intensity of the light that will come forth from the vision that you are about to manifest to the world.

## the mid-wife

In the hour of travail, there is one faithful stalwart in the Kingdom that can be called on to stand by the birthing bed and coach us through the push and pain—the spiritual mid-wife.

A seasoned individual who has either been through the birthing process or walked with so many others that their name is written in the multitude of Kingdom Baby Books: "Aunt Martha: the first one to hold little Pookie;" "Miss Anna: when daddy passed out she kept momma steady, and helped me push you out."

The mid-wife is first a coach, who understands the psycho/spiritual and metabolic changes that one goes through the days, hours and very minutes before they are about to push a big thing though a little space.

They are not afraid of the irrational cussing and screaming in the moment of travail; or of observing the pain seen in the clenched fists and grinding teeth due to the agonizing press that takes place as the vision is squeezed out, while the parent wonders why what started as a night of intimacy ended in a moment of infamy.

The mid-wife is the one that keeps the parent focused in the hour of travail and encourages one to flow with the contractions and breathe between, and push when its time to push; and will know at the moment when one wants to give up the most for fear of passing out that one needs to put the final press and grunt and scream to get what has been on the inside for oh, so long—to get it out!

---

The expectation surrounding this day of revealing, the hour of the birth of vision has been electric.

Those who for years have seen the potential inside of you—your friends and fellow citizens in the Kingdom; your family members whose heart's beat with that of the Beloveds; the needy, broken soul who lives at the end of the block—all who have been awaiting the arrival of your baby are standing outside in the waiting room wanting to see the joyous birth of the vision.

You grab the mid-wife's hand and push, and breath some, and push some more. She says that this is going to be an easy birth, if you ebb and flow with the contractions.

You stare at her in utter amazement, biting your tongue and knowing that if she wasn't holding your hand, it might be inclined to punch her in the face. Can't she see the look of utter contortion on your face and the pressure on you in ways you have never experienced heretofore?

You press some more. In an act of spiritual encouragement the mid-wife prays with you and for you, as you push; from your lips you yell out the name of the baby's father: "Jesus!"

You cry out in the first pangs of travail for the expectation to be revealed: the one that has so gripped you and consumed your inner being until you knew that your destiny was inextricably wrapped up in its seed of powerful potential.

"It's near," says the mid-wife, "Keep your focus on the fruit of your loins and not the fight of faith to bring it forth."

The minutes of what was supposed to be a short birth seem to drag on throughout the evening. Yet somehow in the moment of greatest exhaustion, when there is no energy to pray another syllable, comes the final moments of travail.

In one last push and agonizing cry, the child you have carried is finally squeezed and pressed through the spiritual birth canal and first a head, then upper torso, and finally tiny buttocks and legs plop out into the loving arms of the midwife.

You soon see that the midwife is second a person of great faith.  The world changing potential of your vision is only a slimy, wrinkled little mass of flesh that is still attached to you by a lifeline forged through the months of prayer and gestation in the womb.

In its current state, your baby is not ready to conquer the world, minister to the homeless or care for the helpless. In fact, it can barely lift its head or open its eyes.

But to the mid-wife that doesn't matter.  She sees the great potential of the scrawny vision with the eyes of the Beloved; and cuts the cord, cleans the slime off the child, makes sure all the parts are in place, that its eyes can open and somewhere in the process give the thing a big whack across the back-side; helping the little one to get its first breath of the atmosphere outside the protected place it so recently called home.

---

The birthing of your baby was inevitable.  No matter how much you liked the feel of carrying potential around in your belly it was impossible to keep a growing, already big thing within a small place for too long.

The birth pangs came when the vision was on the verge of getting too big to be pushed out. When the pangs are ignored, either the birth parent or the child will suffer potential damage or death from the effects of vision that is allowed to gestate beyond the appointed hour.

Or the child will be born with birth defects and retardation because they were kept in the place of pressure for too long—the labor pains and travail not responded to in adequate prayer and the child left gasping for breath in the once safe place that became a place of suffocation.

The vision was never intended to stay inside; the world awaits its birth, and its growth will only begin as it is allowed to take those first life-giving breaths of oxygen outside the womb.

## the place of the birth

Mary did not have a choice of where her baby would be born.  Due to the government dictate that all individuals return to their home region to count for the tax, Joseph and she had to return to Bethlehem.

Mary had to endure either a very long hike, or if Joseph's pocketbook agreed a donkey ride through the desert in the ninth month of her pregnancy. She did not have the option of waiting behind and letting Joseph make the trip alone.

In the hour of her greatest discomfort, where the child within was plump, heavy and kicking at the sides of her womb, she had to straddle a beast of burden, endure the rocking and bouncing of the transport sans shock absorbers and the discomfort of riding through the sand, sun and wind of the desert environ.

Had the ass jolted she might have been flung off the beast, water bursting and child delivered in a local gully or oasis, or perhaps miscarried through the injury of the journey.

Mary was not able to birth her child in a place that was comfortable to her or pleasing to her taste for comfort, but in a strange and uninviting land.

None of the older women of the family, Elizabeth, or any of the village mid-wives could make the journey with her. Her first child, born without the warmth of a matronly presence, without the wisdom of experienced birth-mothers and the relative comfort afforded when surrounded by those who knew how to attend to a birth parent's needs.

When Joseph and Mary arrived in Bethlehem, all the available housing, at least the hotel room accommodations of the better quality of the day, were full.

The town was already packed with its returned citizens and there was no room for them in any of the inns. Was it not for the hospitality afforded them to use one of the innkeeper's animal shelters: a barn or cave behind one of the inns, Mary would have had to birth Jesus on the street or in a secluded back alley.

Mary not only had no choice in the geographic place where she birthed her baby, but was totally out of control in the level of comfort, and of those who surrounded her and her family in the nativity hour.

Not only were the women most likely to help her through this first labor not present, but after suffering the long journey on the back of a beast, she had to settle for the only place available that would afford her privacy, minus the inn's animals, in the stall.

---

Like Mary we cannot choose the people or the place where we birth. If the Beloved closes all the doors to the inns in our life and makes sure that the bodies of others are genuinely filling their beds, yet opens a door for us in a barn or cave, is it not His will?

We can complain, cross our arms and pout, but the truth is that when we opened our womb to Him, we gave Him the right to be the father of the thing and the father knows exactly where we need to be before our water breaks.

We may desire a certain level of comfort and conditions that are within our control or cultural proclivities, but the Beloved knows where our child is needed and where to send us to do the hard work of birthing.

We must not fail to see that the barn is merely a birthing center and that we need to make the most of comfort in a strange place. If we are sent to a barn, sweep the floor, put fresh hay in the  manger for the baby, push the farm animals over in the corner and birth the baby.

Conversely, we cannot choose the people that our child will touch.  All, from the unsavory shepherds to the sophisticated kings attended Jesus' nativity and early childhood; and later in life He touched the outcast and poor more often than the rich and refined.

We may steer our child in a direction of caring for the needs of one group only to have the Beloved send us that person or people that doesn't quite fit, or strains our self-image of respectability and cultural dignity.

If our child was born in a barn or cave, let it never forget in the hour of promotion before great men that it was born in hay, surrounded by dung, wrapped in rags and attended to by some of the most salt-of-the-earth type people of the day.

We may walk with our vision among the halls of greatness of the kingdoms of men, but we must never become too great in our own eyes that we cannot touch the people from the place where the vision was born.

# preparing for the arrival

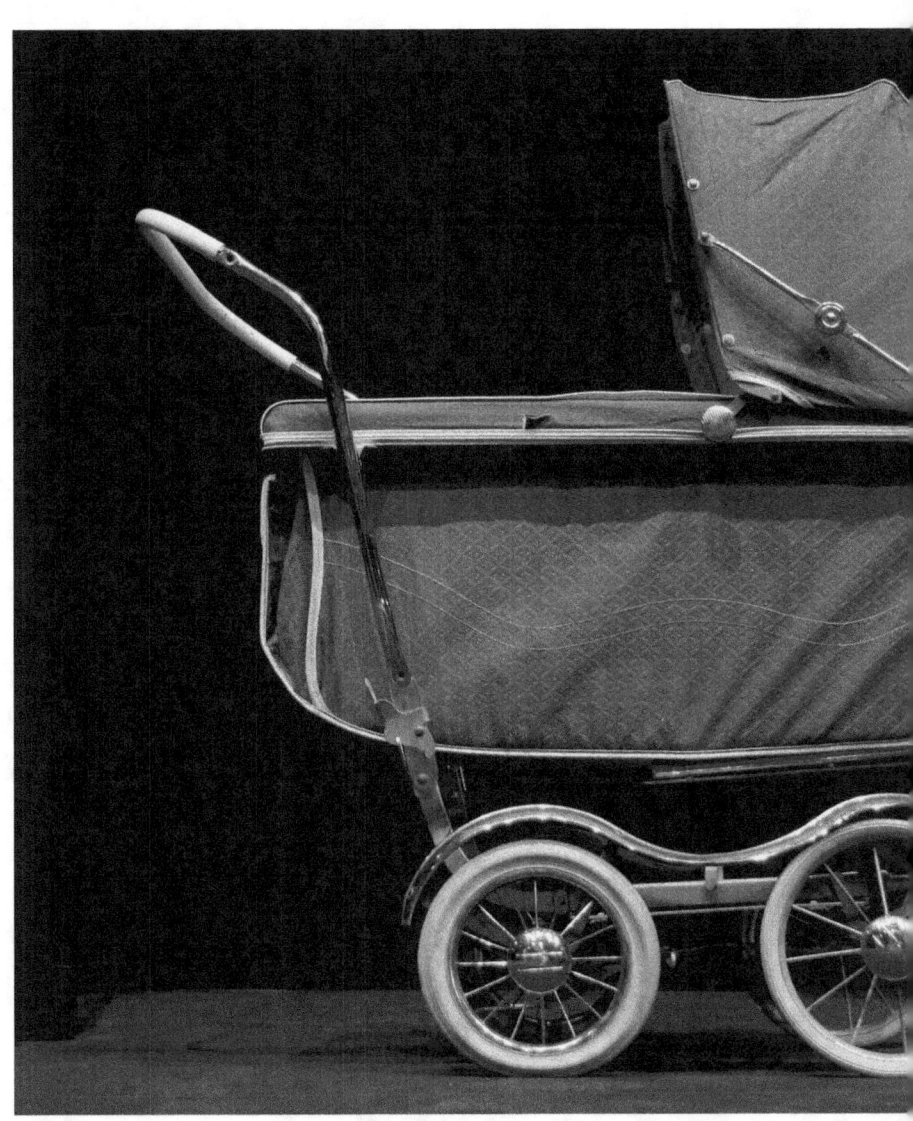

# nanny 911!

There is one individual that is crucial to the success of sustaining the vision you birth: the nanny.

He/she is the Kingdom caregiver—the administratively gifted individual who has the requisite skills and experience to ensure that all preparations are made for the child's appearing.

They are the one who is intimately acquainted with the initial days and years in the life of a vision and instinctively know what to do to make certain the child survives and thrives.

The nanny's role in the Kingdom is twofold: first to make every preparation within the environment that will greet the arrival of your vision, and be its home during its formative years.

And two: to take that which you push out into reality and carefully arrange that the proper nutrition, sanitation and attention is given to the young child so that in time its organizational foundation and infrastructure can support the greatness that is to come.

A well trained nanny has the requisite transferable skills to understand the foundational needs of every child. It does not matter the eventual size, color or complexity that the child will become in time, nor the focus and scope of its outreach.

A good nanny recognizes that the full-grown vision from one womb will look different than that from another, but that there are certain basic needs that must be met in the life of every new-born vision to ensure the success of that vision.

The best nannies, through years of experience, know exactly what infrastructure and systems must be in place in the nursery; know the attention and care that every new-born baby requires; the unique attention to health and nutrition that will need to be present during the early years of development; and understand that every new-born vision in-evitably consumes lots of resources and makes many messes.

## preparation of the nursery

The little room was a flurry of activity. Delivery persons and carpenters vied to complete their varied tasks within the confines of the new nursery.

Over in one corner a group assembled a crib, attaching the side panels, inserting the mattress and other side padding to keep the baby from banging its head on the wooden frame.

In a second corner other workmen constructed a changing table: a waist high flat surface with a padded top, and side drawers that could hold multiple sanitary products and fresh linens.

The air in the room smelled of fresh paint and wallpaper paste; the proof of such seen in the brightly colored walls and the preprinted boarder with baby-themed motifs hung around the ceiling and in a second swath near the chair rail mid-way up the wall from the floor.

With a glance around the room, the baby-themed motif was noted not only in the boarder art, but in the light socket and switch covers, and in the framed posters stacked in a corner waiting to be attached to the wall.

---

The nanny moved gracefully in, about and around the various groups of workers, giving instruction on new tasks and comment on finished work.

She knew that the nursery was the environment that was the key to ensure that the newly birthed vision would be able to survive its early years and thrive as it grew to independence.

If the nursery was well stocked with what the baby needed, there was a greater chance that it would grow to maturity.

As a wise nanny, she understood that the decorative aspect of the nursery—although more desirable than the simple unadorned nurseries of the earlier years of her service—was not the most important aspect of the room.

Certainly, the adornments gave the appearance that this was the room of a new-born, and tickled the fancy of the birth parent and any visitors that might drop in for a visit but it was in no way the intent of this room to be only cute or pretty.

Nanny knew that a nice place for the vision to initially grow was an empty chamber if the substance of the vision was not in place.

She knew that the functions that would take place in the room were not dependent on the attractiveness of the surroundings, but more conditioned on the attentiveness of the care-giver to the needs of the vision and their ability to provide the vision with the required ingredients at the appropriate time.

---

Not only was the room filled with furniture and some pleasing decorative features, but up on the ceiling were a couple rows of small hanging lights connected to moveable tracks, on the floor was a lamp near a strong wooden rocking chair, and on the edge of the changing table was a ceramic lamp in the same baby-themed motif as was in the paper boarder and socket covers.

Nanny was pleased that the room was well lit. She reached over to the wall switch and with a couple quick flicks of the wrist turned the lights on and off.

For the vision to grow properly she knew that it would have to be bathed in light. No baby vision would develop properly in the dark.

Without light nanny would never be able to see the messes or where there were infections attempting to attach themselves to the child.

Nanny sighed as she recalled a vision whose parent refused to develop their baby in the light. Nanny was good at her job, and it didn't take long for her to sniff out the first appearance of messes; there was nothing worse than smelling the mess but not having the light to see where the mess was, and of course not being able to effectively clean up the mess.

That parent's reluctance to grow their vision up in light eventually left the child lying in its own strategic excrement and bedsores that took it to its death.

And, all the while, the parent walking in a state of denial; believing that their child was healthy, growing and prospering, despite the fact that they refused to turn on the light to size up the true condition of their fragile new-born vision.

———————————————————

Also, on the changing table, there was an intercom: the communication system, which would allow the parent or nanny to be able to hear and respond expeditiously to the movements and needs of the new-born.

No vision could long survive without an effective communication system.

If the components of the vision, the care-takers that would come and go from the vision's life and the parent did not have the lines of communication laid, and the appropriate tools and language to communicate, the needs of the child could go unmet for longer than health would allow.

## nutrition and sanitation

The nanny took a seat in the rocking chair in the corner of the nursery. She reached for a small note pad and pencil in her bag on the side of the chair and began to rock back and forth, as her thoughts focused on the final steps in preparing for the arrival of the new vision.

Every so often she stopped rocking, tapped the pencil tip on her pad and scratched a few notes in a script only legible to nannies, health care professionals and other care givers.

In her years as a nanny she had established many nurseries and welcomed numerous new-born visions with well thought out strategies, goals and implementation plans. She instinctively knew the main categories of need that the child would have immediately upon entering the world.

As she compiled her notes, her mind began to race faster than the scribbling on her pad. Turning to a clean page in her notebook she began to organize her thoughts into a more formal list.

The first topic she wrote down was a **proper diet**. A new vision, she recalled, needs a very easy to digest, high protein diet— either the mother's milk or quality bottle formula.

Of course, from her experience, there was no argument that the mother's milk was the best option—as the life flow from the birth parent to the child ensured that the child received the full benefits from the one whose DNA they carried.

Food from any other source could not adequately ensure that the parent's life flow would be transferred to the fledgling vision.

The nanny knew that over time the diet would change, but in the early years of formation, keeping the vision as close to the breast of the parent was the most beneficial: the life giving milk from the founder's tit being the drink that was most suited to strengthen the skeletal structure and the development of the organs and limbs of the child.

---

The nanny leaned back in the chair and proceeded to rock some more, looking around at the nursery that had been so lovingly and professionally laid out only days before.

Over in the corner she noticed the changing table. Turning to another fresh page, the second major point she scribbled on her note pad was **sanitation**. She knew all too well that in the early years, a vision will need its messes cleaned up in a sanitary and discrete fashion.

Every young vision is bound to make some messes—these are not mistakes in the sense that they disqualify one from future development, but are more the natural result of a healthy vision that is experiencing growth and development.

The key to the affect of their messes on the young vision is the response of others to the mess. A nanny must learn to respond in a timely fashion when the scent of mess is in the air. The situation must be sized up, cleaned up, sanitized, powered and perfumed.

The timely, clean-up of messes in the early years keeps the vision from becoming repugnant in the eyes, and noses, of others in the Kingdom. Removing the offending mess also keeps the child from infections that can spread and in time contaminate the whole of the vision.

A sanitary cleaning and disposal of the offensive matter will allow the child to continue to develop as the Beloved intends.

The nanny must have an acute discernment of the needs of the vision, and be willing to make quick assessment of the child's need, and respond to that need in order.

Where some aspect of the vision is making unnatural noise, crying out for attention, or behaving in some other fashion that brings undue attention to itself, the nanny needs to be there.

Once the need is assessed as nourishment, sanitation or weariness, the nanny can respond accordingly, or report the need back to the birth-parent.

## disease and health

The nanny once more leaned back in the chair, not rocking forward but leaning back looking up at the expansive space directly below the ceiling. On another page in her notebook she began to scribble the third main point: **disease and health**.

The nanny thought back to other visions that had been placed under her charge, remembering the vulnerability of the new-born to illness.

Illness, she reasoned, came from outside contaminants that attacked the vision, attempting to enter the body through a weak structure, or uncovered parts of the organization.

Nanny understood that a new-born vision is completely dependent on the care-givers to strengthen their health and protect them from disease. An infection in a weak vision can take the child out within weeks or months following birth.

Worse, an infection can permanently damage the developing structure of a vision, causing the young child to grow up a cripple: growth and development forever stunted; a vision with enough life to be considered viable, but no hope of reaching their potential.

To protect the new born vision, the nanny would have to pay special attention to the parts that were not functioning at normal strength, where inadequate staff, policies or planning could leave the vision open to attack from forces outside or within that did not have the best interests of the child at heart.

Nanny would make sure that all the vulnerable parts of the vision were covered except for the regular cleaning and care that would take place in the privacy of the protected nursery.

Yes, the nursery would be the place where the baby could be isolated, or better insulated from airborne disease: the words and passing comments of others that fly through the airwaves with the goal to infect and contaminate the fresh vision with doubt and death, keeping it from fully developing before it ever had the chance to leave the crib.

Nanny was up to the task and well-prepared to see the child remain contaminate free.

Nanny took each of the main points that she had carefully written in her notebook. Under each topic she compiled a list of tasks that needed accomplishing to support the point, the timeframes to complete each task to be prepared for the arrival of the baby in the nursery, and the supplies that needed to be purchased.

Where other human help was desired to complete one of the details on her list, nanny wrote down a couple namesof individuals who would be qualified to assist.

To the far right of each of her tasks or purchases, nanny estimated a cost.  There were diapers, baby-wipes, antiseptic spray and other supplies to purchase, and she had decided to call on the expertise of a couple of individuals who could assist in monitoring the health of the new-born.

Nanny knew it took money to care for even the smallest of visions.  She totaled up her proposed budget for meeting the child's early needs, rechecked her list and figures, and inserted the document in an envelope addressed to the birth parent.

Before the baby ever entered the nursery nanny wanted to be sure the birth-parent clearly understood the cost of the vision's care.

# the nurture and growth of the child

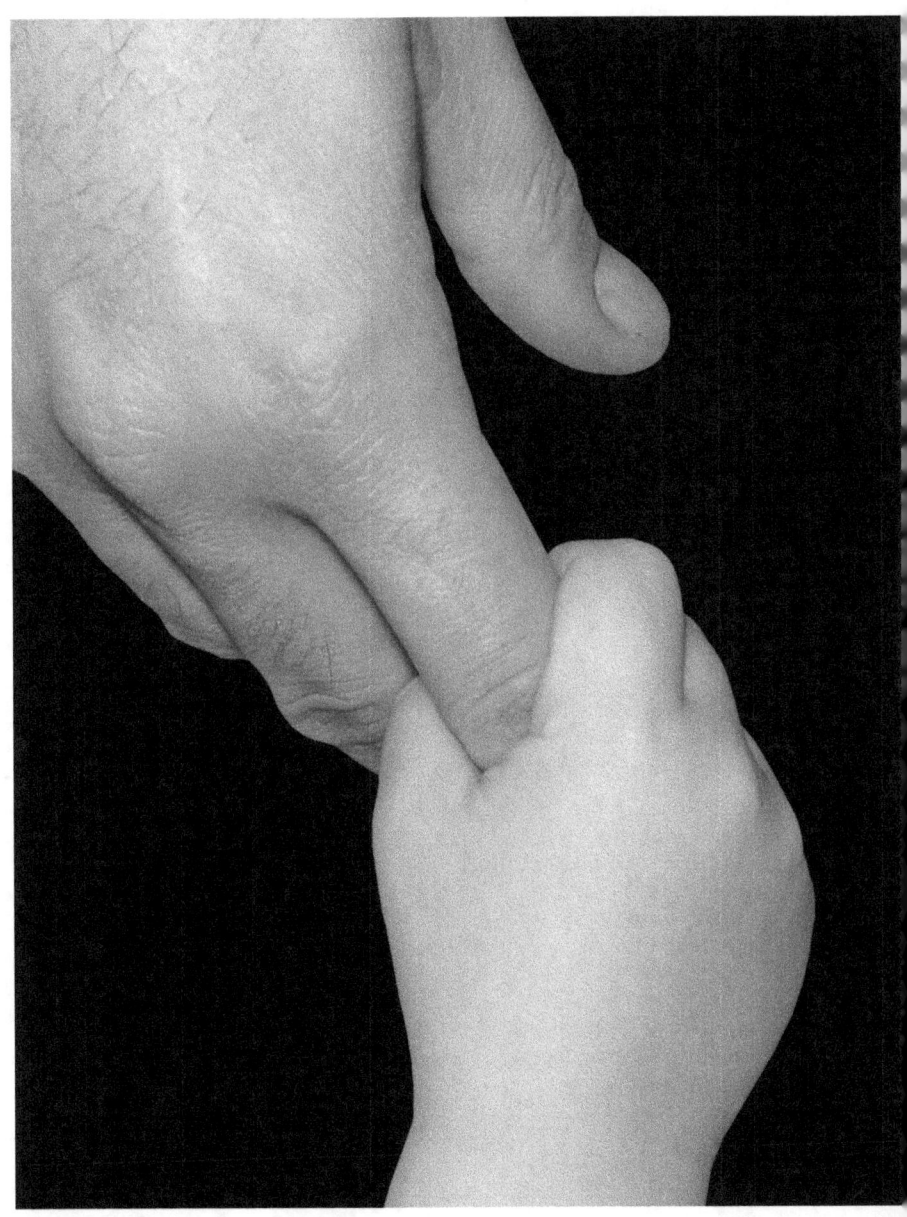

## bringing order

The nanny and the birth parent looked at each other with a big grin. The little baby had made a significant step in its early development.

After weeks of training and prompting the child had toddled over to the small plastic potty, climbed up on its own accord and tinkled, all without the assistance or direction of the two adults.

Once the sound of spray against plastic ceased, the nanny and parent burst out in such applause and verbal praise that one would have though the little vision had won a great award.

In truth the event was a significant sign that the developing vision was maturing; where the vision has the ability and begins to control their own internal functions and if necessary can clean up their own messes.

The adults knew that they would never be able to release the small vision into the public eye without such self-control.

In the history of the Kingdom there had been many visions who were big babies, impressive in size and development, but unable to manage their internal affairs and prone to make messes that stunk up the Kingdom and others had to clean up.

The goal of the care-givers was that the vision would get to the place where they no longer needed to be as acutely attuned to the gurgling, grunts and the passing odors and dampness on the underside that signal that the child is weighed down with a heavy load.

The result of the success of this goal was that the care-givers would no longer be the primary agents of cleaning up the messes. Nanny and the birth-parent knew that:

**A vision that begins to understand how it functions on the inside—and knows how to eliminate strategic waste without fanfare—is a vision that is prepared to move outside of the nursery into greater contact and influence with other Kingdom citizens.**

The independence of the vision had been a theme that was seen in other key events over the prior few months. Long before the potty came into the picture, the vision learned how to be mobile.

It began by rocking and rolling in the crib and on the floor, to the day when the fore-arm and leg strength were enough that the little thing began to pull itself across the nursery floor.

And then one day, when nanny least expected it, the vision stood on its feet and took its first step. Oh, it didn't go far, but the fact that the vision was discovering the world around it and the tools that it had to move in and relate to that world was an eventful stage in its development.

---

Nanny and the birth-parent knew there were other key areas, besides walking and potty-training, where the child would need to develop in order to reach maturity.

One of those areas dealt with eating: the vision taking in the information and human resources which provide nourishment and produce strength.

Eating was a multifaceted change. It involved multiple stages from moving the child from the leader's tit to a bottle; moving from a bottle to solid food; and growing from reliance on others to do the feeding to being able to feed itself.

Keeping the baby close to the breast of the parent is the best way to ensure that the DNA of the parent is passed to the fledgling vision.

But in circumstances where the birth parent is responsible for multiple visions at one time, it may be necessary to quickly wean the vision off the breast milk of the parent and move toward the bottle.

Bottle food, while a close replication of breast milk, gives similar quality nutrition but can often lack the pure DNA flow of the founder.

The move from breast and bottle to solid food is based on the baby's ability to digest information adequately.

The nutrition taken in will still be monitored by the caregivers, and will need to initially be presented in a density and texture that the child can handle. The child is not yet ready to select a balanced diet nor coordinated enough to use the technology to ingest increased amounts of information.

The parent of a small vision will need to be involved in the feeding of the vision until the day it is able to make its own educated and healthy decisions.

The move to the vision being able to eat solid food, on its own, is another step that will eventually bring it independence. When a vision can monitor the information and diet that it ingests, it can make choices concerning its development without the input of outside sources.

---

A second important area in the vision's development is teaching the child manners and how to interact with other children in the Kingdom of the Beloved and those of men.

While the sanctity of the nursery is a positive environment for the nurture and protection of a vision, it will become a prison if the vision never grows to the place where it can effectively touch the other citizens that it exists for.

And, a vision will misrepresent the birth parent and/or the Beloved if it violates the rules, roles and respect that are expected to be exhibited outside the atmosphere of the nursery.

The vision needs to understand that increasing levels of professional growth and spheres of influence require increasing levels of responsibility.

The rules of the nursery are a good foundation for life in the Kingdom, but the actual interaction with others in the Kingdom of the Beloved and those of men will involve learning to interpret those simple nursery rules to a myriad of personalities and complexity of interactions.

The foundation of the rules will always be what was taught in the first years of the vision, but will be reinvented and communicated based on the level of sophistication of the situation at hand.

## teaching stewardship

To raise a child to steward its own future and destiny appropriately, the parent and care-givers need to understand the unique gifting and calling of the vision. A vision cannot be expected to grow up to take care of itself if it is not properly cared for by the adults who are initially at it side.

The questions that affect gifting and calling include: What are the strengths and weaknesses of the vision; what is the temperament of the vision, and where and how will the vision function in the Kingdom?

Each vision will have its unique strengths and weaknesses. These are usually formed in uterus although they can be developed following delivery through the influence of others.

A vision that is properly thought out during development will have the greatest chance of being birthed with a strong structure and support. But, a vision that is not strategically thought out while swimming in the womb may come into the world with built in structural defects.

Where the administrative nanny is not consulted early in the life of such a vision, the structural defects will keep the vision from healthy growth.

---

The birth parent had heard of a vision born in a neighboring nursery. The parent of that child was overjoyed at carrying the Beloved's seed, but failed to think through what it meant to birth a vision, and through ignorance failed to call on one of the well-trained local nannies.

The joy over the birth overshadowed the need for practical planning.

The vision was born, and in time appeared to develop as it grew in the number of activities it encompassed and personnel that attended its needs, but due to foundational structural weakness, the pressure of additional programs and personnel caused the structure to buckle under the weight.

At the point that the structure failed a nanny was hired, who through months of painful manipulation of staff and resources rescued the vision from the dust-bin of poorly thought out ideas.

---

No child can ever get to the place of stewarding itself without a clear understanding of its strengths and weaknesses. Nor can a vision be fully developed without understanding its temperament.

Nanny knew that a vision's temperament will usually reflect that of the birth-parent.  Where the temperament of the founder is compassionate the vision will be warm and inviting toward the hurting and homeless; where the vision's mission is forceful and prophetic, resisting tyranny and oppression, the birth-parent is usually the same.

The need to understand temperament is kin to knowing the place and how the vision will function; prophetic may not be helpful to the one who needs compassion and warmth while undiscerning concern may lack respect among the prophetic.

The place and the people the child is called to serve will depend on the need and the unique call that the child can meet.  The Beloved knows that need before the birth, and forms in the womb the one who will be used to specifically meet that need.

Proper understanding of who the child is and will become is crucial to keep the caregivers from moving beyond the influence the vision will have or resources of people and money that are allocated to the vision; a breach of which could potentially endanger the work or raise false expectations in others that the vision would ultimately be unable to meet.

When the caregivers understand the sphere of influence that the vision is called to and the resources that are present to walk out the vision, they can place increasing expectations and responsibility on the vision.

The adequate time and attention given to the newborn will then diminish over time as the vision develops and moves towards increasing independence

## utilizing outside resources

The type of vision and its level of maturity, and the skill level and knowledge of the caregivers will determine if there is a need to bring in outside resources to strengthen the vision.

When, in the vision's development, it is noticed that there is a deficiency in the child's progress; it is here that the skills and influence of another is necessary: Kingdom Consultants, coaches and confidants; tutors, teachers and trainers—others from outside that are brought in to teach and instill key principles or actions in the vision.

Discerning deficiencies is directly related to the long-term plans that you have for the child.

If he/she is to grow up in a certain sphere of influence, or if there are expectations that they will perform a specific skill or service, and it is noted that amidst the growth and development of the baby there is a lack—that is where the services of another must be called on.

Calling in the outside provider is not a sign of inability on the part of the care-givers. In fact, it is the opposite: a sign of their sensitivity and discernment of where the child is vs. where it needs to be.

It is the poorly qualified care-giver that misses the fact that the vision is not developing on time.  The nanny who lacks experience or discernment can miss the signs of an underdeveloped vision.

Some nannies, fearful of admitting their lack of skill and training, determine that they are the only one with the requisite skills and prowess to influence the child, and thereby become threatened by the input of others.

When a better trained nanny offers their observations on the child's development, they will be silenced.

Silencing other's contributions will limit the growth of vision, and potentially suffocate the child—especially when the intimidated nanny is overbearing and holds an incomplete understanding of the vision's needs.

---

Outside resources are especially beneficial when investing in health giving exercises—an annual check-up—such as an organizational assessment that serves to see if the vision is functioning in a healthy manner.

In high-maintenance and understaffed visions, the caregivers can easily loose perspective on the actual condition of the child.

The analysis and input of a trained outsider places the realities of the experience of the vision against the original mission and goals the vision was birthed to fulfill.

Where the reality and the mission mirror each other, the baby is healthy—where one or the other do not reflect each other, there is a need to either align the realities back up with the mission, or reevaluate the mission in light of the dissonance.

Once the Kingdom consultant or coach has helped the caregivers with the assessment of the vision, they can make recommendations and set a plan to return the vision to the place of organizational health.

## babies first day out

The vehicle of choice was an old-fashioned perambulator or "pram": a miniature carriage-type vehicle sitting on four sizeable metal-spoke wheels, with a moveable cover to protect from the sun, and a raised bar at the rear used to push and steer the contraption.

The occasion was the first time the small vision would be taken out of the protected nursery and be presented in public.

In preparation, the nanny took the little vision and gently placed it in the bottom of the pram, all surrounded by cushions and a few of baby's favorite play things.

Nanny knew that the first time out in public in the pram should be a grand affair.

Most, except the inner circle, will not have seen the new vision. While there may have been the occasional photograph and the verbal announcement sent to say that the child was birthed, few have actually seen the flesh and blood thing that they have waited patiently for.

Nanny also knew that the roll-out of the child should be executed to draw much attention.

It was important to roll it out when the child was most alert, and able to respond to the direct tactical influence of passersby as a vision that was dull or listless would leave a mixed impression.

It was also key to put on the best clothes, shoes, ribbons in the hair, and wrap the baby in a soft blue or pink blanket, depending on what kind of vision the child was.

---

On the way out the door, nanny stopped to think through the route she, the pram and the wee vision should take.

She thought, "The roll-out of the vision should be among those who have been already adequately prepped that a new vision was being birthed, and that the time to publicly parade the baby had come.

Those who have heard about the vision and are eagerly expecting its appearance will be attracted to the pram and other finery that clothe the child."

The nanny reasoned that she should definitely spend the day walking down paths where those who have been expectantly waiting the child reside.

If they are in the lane of the park, in midday, be there; if they are in the church-hall at night, show up; wherever those who will most likely have a favorable response to the birth of the vision are, that is where you want to be.

As she pushed the pram down the carefully chosen lanes, first one then another of the Kingdom denizens stopped their conversations and other outing activities to come and take a look at the new vision.

"My, my," said one older man, "it is a fine plan, with a strong infrastructure and so appealing too!"

Another woman, an older mother in the Kingdom, stopped to take a peak, pinch the cheeks of the baby and nodded her head in approval: "You'll grow to be a find organization, won't you," she said, as she took her leave.

All in all, by the time the nanny walked the planned circuit and returned to the nursery, only a few passersby stopped to even look at the child.

"Not to worry," she said to the little bundle in the pram. She knew all too well from her years of experience that a child's influence initially extended only to the handful of people in their small world.

But, it was those few people who were the beginning of a ripple effect that would take the news of the fresh vision far and wide.

Nanny knew that as the chosen handful see the baby, begin to understand the child's potential, pinch its pudgy little cheeks, and "Ooh" and "Aah" and "Koochee Coo" over the plans for its future; they will soon take their delight and share it with their friends and family, and pretty soon there will be an ever expanding network of those who think the vision is the greatest most influential thing to ever come down the Kingdom lane.

———————————————————————

Recently, nanny had returned to school to be trained in media and the internet.

She reasoned that these new tools would be seen as not only an asset in this day and age, but in some circles a requirement for her to remain a savvy, employable nanny.

But, even after lengthy training she began to see that the pram still worked best with the initial and immediate circle of influence.

While many parents posted the picture of their new-born vision on the web for all their friends and multiplied others to see, its influence went no further then the prams; attracting the attention of only a small circle of influence.

Any strangers, surfing the web, who happened to click on an image of the vision would not be initially impressed with the baby; remember it is small, wrinkled and perhaps half-bald and many will not see the potential in the child as you or your staff do.

Time will be necessary for your little thing to be impressive enough to sell itself over the internet or the airwaves.

The public will have to see your vision in a number of different formats, or be directed to it by the immediate circle of well-wishers before it will exert any great influence on the masses in the ether world.

Before the multitudes ever acclaim your vision, it will likely have to exert an influence on many smaller groups and audiences of one, and probably be lived out in an obscure place before the thing makes its way before the great.

# releasing the child

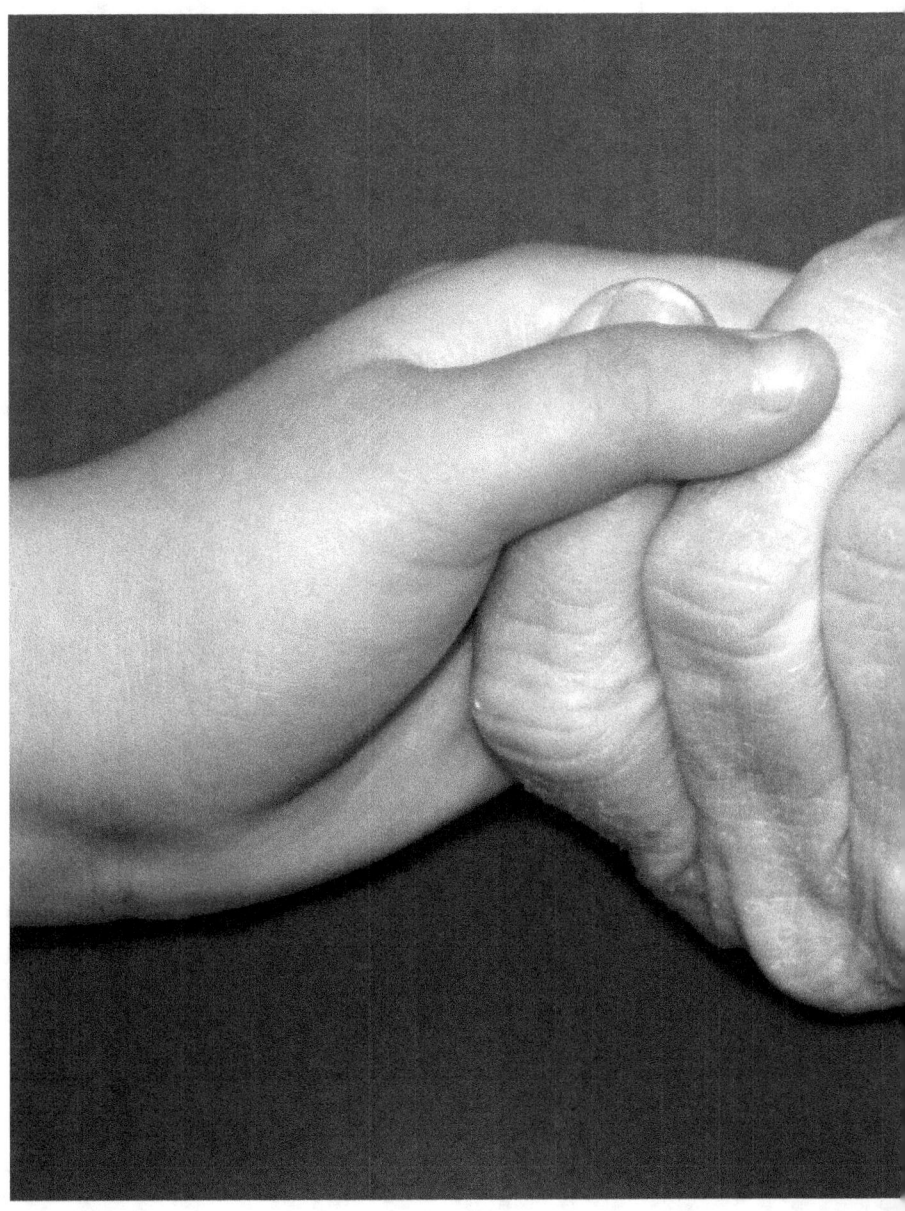

# letting go of the vision

In the development of every child, a season arrives when it moves from utter dependence on the birth parent to a place of increased independence.

A child so recently tender and vulnerable is growing in their ability to make decisions affecting their present circumstances, and is even beginning to chart their own course in life.

Significant to this transition is the fact that the parent is not as necessary to the child's survival as in the early years, their role having diminished over time and been replaced by that of other mentors and peers. The child is grown.

A vision follows a similar cycle from dependence to independence. The vision you carried, birthed and lovingly tended to for years has grown to the place where your role is changing significantly if not coming to an end.

You took care that the nannies were in place and the nursery was stocked with formula, diapers, warm clothes and toys; you ensured that the growing years were filled with suitable influences in teachers and other companions.

You carried the primary weight of responsibility for the vision through good times and turmoil, peace and heartache.

In a scenario whose existence you either dreaded or denied, you wake up one morning to the awareness that the thing that you birthed so many years before has now grown well beyond your initial expectations.

And, you instinctively realize that your season of influence in the process of the vision's development is complete.

Of course, you could linger around longer, but as your input into the daily care of the vision has waned to a somewhat emeritus role, your purpose in the next season of the child's development is negligible.

In the life of a vision there inevitably is a season where the one who birthed the vision must move off the scene so that the child can grow, through the influence of others, beyond the capacity and limitations of the birth parent.

This is never an easy prospect or process as the paternal/maternal instinct in most is strong. We agonized over and nurtured the child for so long that we cannot conceive that we would ever find ourselves in the position where we no longer play a vital or influential part in the vision's development.

How could we who carry the DNA of the vision, and instinctively recognize the meaning of every movement and hiccup of the child relinquish our role as caregiver?

Even though the vision is strong and mature, how can it survive without our daily influence?

In truth, the vision will survive, and should the proper support be put in place before your departure, the minds of those who also carry the vision's DNA will be able to grow it to a depth of strength and maturity that was not previously conceivable.

---

Letting go of a vision is difficult because in many our identity is reflected in the vision we birthed—we are known by the child at our side.

When we walk down the lanes of the Kingdom it is our child that usually brings the attention and delight of pass-ersby.

While, out of cultural custom, they cordially greet us, it is the plump freshness and influence of our child that will cause them to stoop and pinch and tickle with delight. They see the potential and influence in our offspring and complement us on the healthiness of our vision.

When the child is no longer at our side our identity is lost. While the crowds were once drawn to see our baby, they are amazingly not so interested in seeing us without the world-changing, Kingdom-influencing one who we could once claim as our own.

It is not that their respect for our role in the Kingdom, or admiration for our character and calling has changed. But, without the viable, fresh presence of the child at our side, we loose the one that became the natural ice breaker for multiple conversations.

Even if we have suitably separated our sense of identity and self-worth from our vision, and we understand how critical it is for the further growth and development of the vision that we relinquish our control over it; it is still a hard thing to let go of a child.

The investment of time, energy, wealth and flesh, sweat and blood that have been poured into the development, protection and survival of our offspring can never be regained.

Our vision was a piece and part of who we are, and although our influence over daily needs will fade, it will always remain a reflection of the one who gave it life.

## moving off the scene

The feeling had grown inside for some time; input and direction into the vision that I once perceived was counted as useful and appreciated had apparently begun to become a nuisance, the topic of frustrated, muttered words under the plastic smiles of others.

The Kingdom caregivers that I put in place and trained continued to patronize me and comply with my directives even though they were fully capable to care for the vision without my input.

The child had grown to the place where, when once he could not go through an hour in a day without my direction, he was now able to survive for long stretches of time without me.

In fact, there were whole weeks where I didn't need to know the details of the operation because the others who I entrusted with the care of the child were more than responsible for his every need, and even surprised me as they responded with wisdom and grace through the odd crises.

Some days, there were moments when I sat on my swivel chair, glanced around at the whole of the nursery and realized that all was running smoothly.

Without my active presence and wisdom there were multiple groups of attendants walking out the vision.

Certainly the occasional question would be directed my way, and I would spin my chair around in the direction of the Kingdom caregiver, listen intently, rub my forefinger and thumb on my chin in a sign of sagely wisdom and answer the question.

But, despite the occasional question, I was not really needed in the nursery. My time as a caregiver of the one I birthed was coming to a close.

There were other telling signs that a transition was imminent. The months prior to my departure I noticed that not only was I not really necessary to the success of the operation, but that the grace and joy I had experienced in the earlier years of executing the vision had lifted.

I found my attention drifting from the child to other places and pursuits. I even secretly began to fantasize about having another baby; strongly desiring a fresh vision planted in my womb and actually thought longingly about pregnancy and setting up a new nursery for the eventual arrival.

Even through I ultimately knew it was time to move on, emotionally I flipped back and forth between the desire to stay and wanting to move forward.

I found that the Beloved would one day directly challenge me to see if I was willing to move on, and at other times would see if I were willing to stay right were I was.

His prodding and my 'flexible' emotional state put me in a position where I found myself less and less attached to the vision.

My emotional fingers were being slowly pried from off the one I had been responsible for. I was aware that the paternal instinct that runs deep was being challenged to let go.

I mentally understood what the Beloved was doing; detaching me emotionally from the vision so that I could move on, but honestly my cognitive understanding did not help to smooth the emotional process of tearing, grieving, and dieing that I had entered in to.

Many a day I mentally took my Isaac, the child of so much promise up to the mountain, prepared wood for the altar and raised my knife to slew the child, only to find that unlike the biblical narrative there was no ram in the thicket.

The Beloved was not testing me to see if I would theoretically kill my child; but was demanding that I take the knife and sever the ties with that child, set fire to the altar and let it burn as a pleasing sacrifice, the smoke of which would ascend before the divine nostrils.

Moving on meant that there was no ram to take the place of the vision; there was only a death to the vision, and a moving off the scene, not knowing what would come next for my child of promise or me.

## entrusting the child to another

There is much to be aware of as a birth parent moving off the scene of a vision. The strategy and timing associated with your exit will determine if your child is able to successfully continue to grow and thrive, or becomes stymied because of the emotional loss of 'you'.

From the moment that you are aware that change is imminent, it is vital to make every preparation for your departure away from the place of authority in the life of the child.

The Beloved would not move you on unless He perceived that the individuals who will take your place were already in the wings waiting for their marching orders.

They are the ones that you trained and entrusted with the intimate functions of the child. Their service to and passion for the baby is evident to all.

But, even where others have faithfully served for long seasons and are prepared to move into greater responsibility, it is necessary to set up the structures that will allow the child to prosper through the transition.

As you hand over the vision entrust it to those who understand and cherish the DNA of the child.

Once in the position of authority they may not do things the same way as you. They will probably add their own unique contributions to the vision over time; but they will not unintentionally kill the child by dressing it in clothes that do not fit, pushing it out into activities that it is not suited for or violating the foundational mission that is core to the child's existence.

The uniqueness of the vision will look differently, based on the passion and gift-mix of the caretakers that are left in charge. This is good, as they will hopefully build upon the investment and impartation that you poured into the child when you walked with it on a daily basis.

Unfortunately, the vision can be destroyed, suffering an untimely death, if the caretakers do not have the heart to understand the purpose for its existence in the Kingdom for the hour at hand.

---

As you fully relinquish control over the baby, give the others involved in the process time to make the mental and emotional shift.

Upon hearing of your succession plan, those who have walked with you and the child as caregivers may experience simultaneous emotions of both fear and delight: fear over the question of their adequacy to care for the vision without you in the picture; delight at the new challenges and promotion that will come with their need to step to the plate to take your place.

Honor relationships with those who you have served, leave your blessing on the child and the caretakers; and move off the scene.

In the transition, give advise when asked, but don't continue to hover around the child; when you were present in the life of the child it was healthy, but when you are gone, too much of your unneeded presence will make you appear like a stalker, hiding in the shadows, attempting to keep pulse on the vision, and the every movement of the new caregivers.

When you leave, really leave.  If you have to remain physically close to the nursery, step back into the shadows in an emeritus status, staying out of the decision making process for the vision, or only contributing when invited.

Where it is not possible to stay close to the nursery without wanting to lead, put some geographic distance between you and the child.

Verbally affirm the state and health of the vision and the caretakers, and be careful to not grumble and complain when they make decisions about the child's care and growth that are not acceptable to your thought process.

## train up a child in the way they should go

From the first moment that our little vision opens its eyes to the cold world and makes its presence known by a whimper or squeal, we should adamantly follow the biblical injunction and train up that child in the way they should go (Prov 22:6).

The way they should go is a set path through life that will allow them to blossom and become all that the Beloved has intended them to be and do.

Unfortunately, if we have mixed motives, the way our vision should go is often not what we desire.  I may want my baby to be true to me, revere me and obey me all the days of my life, and to develop organizationally in the plans that I strategically laid out at its birth.

I may want my vision to become a monument to my success in the Kingdom. But, despite my desires as the birth parent, the ultimate way the child should go is in a path that the Beloved has set out for them.

**It is during the time a birth parent moves off the scene, in the midst of the emotional sorrow of severing, the sobering reality must be illumined on the conscience of the parent that the vision was never really theirs in the first place.**

As the parent you may have gown to believe that it was the cleverness of your imagination, the maturity of your gift or the force of your character that brought the vision to its present state.

But, like all children, who are a gift from the Beloved, He was the Father of the thing, the vision was planted in your open womb by Him, and you were merely the responsible steward for His child until the day of transitioning off the scene.

Yes, your gifts and skills contributed to the development of the vision and you were a great parent, but the Beloved determines when it is time for you to relinquish your role over that child.

---

Remember Moses' mother. She birthed her baby of promise, fooling the Egyptians, protecting her child from Pharaonic infanticide by putting him in a mud and waddle basket, taking him to the edge of that great flowing, muddy current and letting him float to an uncertain future down the Nile.

She had a very clear understanding, as we all must from day one, that her child was not really hers. When she pushed him off the shore down into the torrent of that crocodile infested river, she had surely turned his fate over to Jehovah.

You know the rest of the story. God graciously sent Pharaoh's daughter to find the basket with its precious cargo, and despite recognizing it as one of the Hebrew's children, bestowed favor on the child in her eyes; she called for Moses' mother to wet nurse and care for the child through its early years.

Moses was never his birth mother's vision. Had she not relinquished her right to control the limits of Moses' potential or the outcome of the story; Moses might have been early on killed even on the birthing stool, or held back from achieving an influence on a national level.

For us as parents, we must discern our place and our season of influence, and graciously move off the scene when our investment is complete.

If we linger around too long, beyond the time appointed by the Beloved, the vision can be constricted by our limitations, cease to grow and even begin to atrophy.

If we obediently move off the scene in the right time the child will continue to experience growth that will be way beyond the limits of our potential, into the limitless potential of the Beloved.

For the birth parent of a vision this will be the second and final time they will have to push their child out: the first time being the pushing out from the protected womb and the cutting of the connection through the umbilical cord; the second and final time at the moment of their child's independence.

If a parent in either season refuses to push or move; the child can be suffocated and will eventually die.

# when a child
# is taken by force

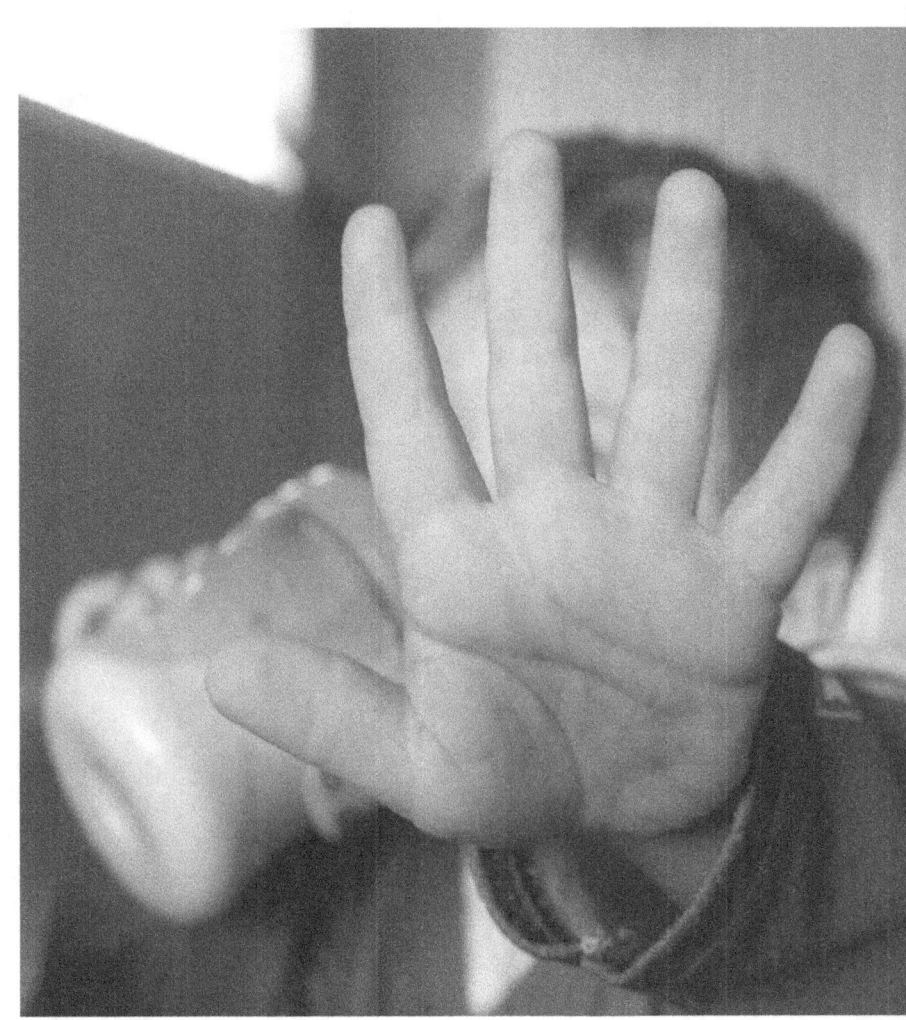

## when favor shifts

The Kingdom Citizen had birthed a child within the protective covering of a larger vision.

Her heart and energies were focused on the nurture and admonition of her baby, knowing that the success of the one named after the larger vision would reflect favorably upon those in whose employ she toiled.

In the midst of her work the Citizen failed to pay serious attention to the winds of change that blew down the hallway of her corner of the Kingdom.

The changes started out slowly, where Citizen noted that routine requests for supplies for the nursery that formerly were always approved were being questioned and denied.

Following a change in management, she began to hear comments from the new powers that were in control that actually questioned the purpose and fruitfulness of the vision, and wondered what the child would look like without its arms and a leg; or, perhaps that it could better serve the Kingdom if the child were killed and a new vision adopted.

In time the suggestions for change accelerated in interval and intensity until Citizen began to take note that even her role as caregiver of the vision was in question.

With the shift in leadership and focus in vision, she asked multiple questions to clarify future direction for her program and understand her role, if any, in the proposed expansion of the vision.

Her questions were essentially useless. There was new leadership in her corner of the Kingdom, and that invisible, but all important component called favor had lifted off of her.

Without favor, Citizen believed that her incessant questioning of the plans and demands of the new leadership put her in a place where she appeared not competent to care for the vision and uncooperative.

At a point when she was told to sever certain limbs and even dissect vital organs from the child, she questioned the decision, knowing full well that the mission and core purpose of the vision would be damaged irreparably, leading to the eventual death of the child.

———————————————————————

Wondering how the favor that had attended the birth and early years of her baby was apparently evaporating, she walked around the hallway for days in a state of shock.

Wasn't the fruit of a multitude of lives strengthened, cared for and fitted for Kingdom service sufficient to support the continued need to resource and grow the vision?

Wasn't the glowing praise of the hundreds of those who had labored by her side an adequate testimony to her fitness as a parent?

In her shock Kingdom Citizen failed to swiftly acknowledge the shifting sands of favor.

Had she judged accurately she might have departed on her own initiative from her caregiver role, but instead she waited in hope that the fruitfulness of her child and the tangible contribution she and the little vision had made to the larger vision were adequate enough to maintain her position.

Her judgments were proved wrong on the sad day that her child was removed from her care; and she removed forever from the role of caregiver.

———————————————————————

It was a scene too often repeated in the Kingdom: a birth parent removed from the direct care of a child.

In transitions that appear sudden and almost without warning the parent is terminated from their position within an organization, or a board of directors determines that it is time for "new blood" to direct the vision.

Within a matter of days or even hours of the decision, the parent is either escorted from the premises of the nursery or finds themselves sipping punch and nibbling peanuts and cake at their fare-well party.

# why did they take my baby?

**It is a hard thing to give up a child on your own accord; it is excruciatingly painful to have a child taken away by force and without warning.**

A birth parent cannot pour their life into the creation, birth, development and health of a fledgling vision; have the child snatched from their care and walk away without bearing some measure of emotional pain.

The pain may range from a numb internal ache to a trail of dripping blood left behind a broken heart; but the pain will be real to the one who has lost the child.

The emotional response to the death of a vision is similar to a physical death in the stages that one has to wander through before reaching a place of sanity and peace.

The manner in which the transition was accomplished determines the level of shock and unbelief that will attend the transition event.

If adequate communication and time were given to digest the change and the ability to say fare-well granted, the initial emotional transition stages will be weakened in their punch. But, as too often is the case, where the timing of the transition is unexpected, the affect on the birth parent is shock and confusion.

---

Even though she observed months of changes that directly affected her ability to care for the vision, Citizen was not prepared to be unceremoniously removed from her role as caregiver.

Her mind and emotions swirled with disbelief at what had just transpired. Her initial thought was that perhaps a mistake was made and maybe the ones in control didn't know about the decision.

Citizen's initial disbelief quickly morphed into reasoning with self that if a mistake was made, perhaps it could be rectified.

She thought that maybe there was something that she could do or say that would cause them to take her back. And that once they recognized their mistake; they would willingly welcome her return to her role as caregiver.

Citizen didn't stay long in the reasoning stage, quickly becoming angry at self for not moving off the scene when she began to note change in the air, and anger at the individuals she perceived took the child.

Over a period of days, Citizen's emotions played out to the most painful final stage of grief and sorrow: the sad realization that it was all over in her relationship to what had once been her pride and joy.

By this stage the shock had worn away, the anger subsided, and through tearful eyes the recognition was finally made that no amount of reasoning, bargaining or plotting would convince those who removed her from her caregiver role to return her to that position.

Grief and sorrow left Kingdom Citizen with a nagging question: was she unfit as a parent to raise the child just taken, and if so, how could she ever think of caring for any other visions that might come her way in future years.

## am I an unfit parent?

It is especially difficult to lose a child with the stigma that you were an unfit parent.

When Child Protective Services knocks at the door of the house where the vision lives, questioning your parenting skills, insinuating that your influence on your child is negative and eventually escorting the child out the door, loading your baby into a white van and driving off into an uncertain future; the result is a deep humiliation.

Once removed from the oversight of your child and the question of your fitness becomes a topic of public consumption, the scales of justice no longer leave you a verdict of innocent until proven guilty—the act of removal tips the scale on the guilty side.

In the public's eye if there were no guilt, then you would still be at your child's side. Little thought is given to the questions of why exactly your child was taken away.

For example, you may have been a completely perfect caregiver to the vision, but as often happens, the voices of those in the Kingdom who do not have the heart of the King whispered in the ears of those with power, casting dispersions on your character and competence, in time eroding the confidence that the leader had in your parental abilities.

You may in fact have been a stellar parent, but another with darker intentions, who desired to become a parent without understanding the heart of a parent, or exhibiting a willingness to conceive and birth their own vision, usurped your position.

Thinking they could take your place as parent, but failing to recognize the cost of parenting, they worked to push you to the side and snatch the custodial rights over the child.

What ever the reasons you were removed from the care of the vision, the result is humiliation and endless unanswered questions.

You may never know why your child was taken. You may be left to years of reasoning with self of what you could have done, or should have avoided.

As you don't know the truth you are left to empty speculative replies to those who ask what happened to your child.

And, sadly, many people will never speak to you again—because they saw your child taken away—but instead of addressing you face-to-face will whisper and speak of you in the dark shadows outside your door.

If your child has been taken, you can never answer or silence all the voices of your humiliation. You can never go back and right  the wrongs or explain the misperceptions that took place before the child was removed from your custody.

If child protective services have visited, and their departure emptied your life of a vision, you will need to ask yourself three hard questions. Whether perception or reality, children are taken for one of the following:

---

*Neglect* – Did you neglect your child? Your interests and focus began to change. You knew transition was imminent, as your joy in the parenting process waned, and you longed for the freshness that you experienced with new vision.

But, in the midst of the change, you were not willing to face the new reality, release authority and control and the child got neglected and suffered in the process.

Needs that formerly were addressed immediately festered like boils, until others took note of the lack of timely care given to the vision.

Perhaps your neglect was reflected in the caregivers and other volunteers that attended the vision.  Did they feel adequately appreciated; were their financial, emotional and professional needs met—or did you fail to see the fatigue on their faces and the verbal hints that they were feeling neglected?

Did you fail to offer clear and decisive leadership when your team began to flounder in the mire of your waning interest in the vision?

Did you miss the chance to further develop the child when fresh opportunity was presented because you didn't want to expend the energy for something that was no longer life-giving to you?

Regardless of your decreasing interest and emotional investment, a growing vision cannot be ignored; it will be fed and nurtured for growth, or it will loose mass and strength and shrink from neglect.  The vision will not take a break in development, circling in a type of holding pattern until you decide that you are once again interested in its future.

---

*Over-indulgence* – Did you overindulge your vision? You made poor decisions on behalf of the child and gave too much unwarranted attention or provision to the thing when it needed discipline and focus.

In your over-indulgence you unwittingly neglected certain aspects of the vision, or the role of the vision in relationship to others in the Kingdom.

Lavish attention devoted to a fat, lazy child does not hide the child's fatness or laziness from the gaze of others. Your fitness as a parent will be questioned if you dote on the vision with sweets when it needs to be exercised.

If you lavished too much time and attention directed to favorite aspects of the vision, while other pieces were left to attend to themselves, your child would begin to appear off balance.

People took note and commented that your child had some obese parts and other emaciated parts in the same body.

As an overindulging parent, you spent too freely: over-committing resources to an already plump child, and thus wasting valuable funding and time that eventually produced lean times for the vision.

---

*Over-possessiveness* – Were you over-possessive when it came to your baby? Perhaps you were not willing to let go of status or control over an older child who had been by your side for years.

Over time, your identity and sense of purpose were so completely wrapped up in the child that you failed to discern and take advantage of the hour of your departure, and stayed around long beyond the point of being welcome.

Or like Kingdom Citizen, perhaps you had a strong sense of loyalty to the broader vision that your child served, and believed that your commitment to the greater good would be valued during organizational transition.

The sad reality is that *misplaced loyalty is idolatry*! When the Beloved calls you forward, you must move even if it means giving up control of the nurture of something you birthed.

For the one called to forward motion who fails to leave in a timely manner, the season will come that he or she will be pushed out the door.

## picking up the pieces

Like a multitude of others throughout Kingdom history, Citizen too spent nights on the edge of her bed, mourning the loss of her child.

But as her emotions played out over the days and weeks, she found the pain receded in intensity. Even the swirl of agonizing thoughts that attended her child's removal eventually seemed a distant echo in her mind.

As she rested, there were two ideas impressed on her mind and spirit. First was the recognition that although the vision had been taken, the Father of the child had not abandoned her.

The organization where she birthed the child had deemed her no longer fit to care for the vision, but the organization was not the vision's father—the Father was still by her side.

Second, she understood that as long as the Beloved was present in her life, and her womb remained open to His touch, she could again conceive, carry and birth other visions.

She knew that once the tears were over and her heart was mended, she would be available and useful again for His good pleasure.

Over the months Citizen rested in her relationship with the Beloved. She let Him touch the insecurity over her capability that had formed around the edges of her heart.

Her heart was not hardened, but she noticed the scabs that covered her former wounds, her insecurities and the sense of being dropped by those she trusted attempted to link together and form a solid crust over her heart.

As she maintained an attitude of trust in the Beloved and forgiveness towards those she perceived dropped her; the scabs and insecurities remained as small islets floating around in a vast sea.

When she allowed herself to slip into bitterness, and pulled away from the presence of the Beloved, the islets quickly linked up until larger land masses formed and became hard over her heart.

To keep her heart soft, she came before the Beloved with more abandon than in any other season in her life.

In the midst of His healing presence she grew less concerned about the vision that was taken, and about the need to birth other visions to appear fruitful before the eyes of others.

Over time, she found her heart healed, motives cleansed and her hands once again empty of future plans. And, somewhere in the midst of the process, the Beloved's presence had once again become her all-consuming desire.

# spiritual player's

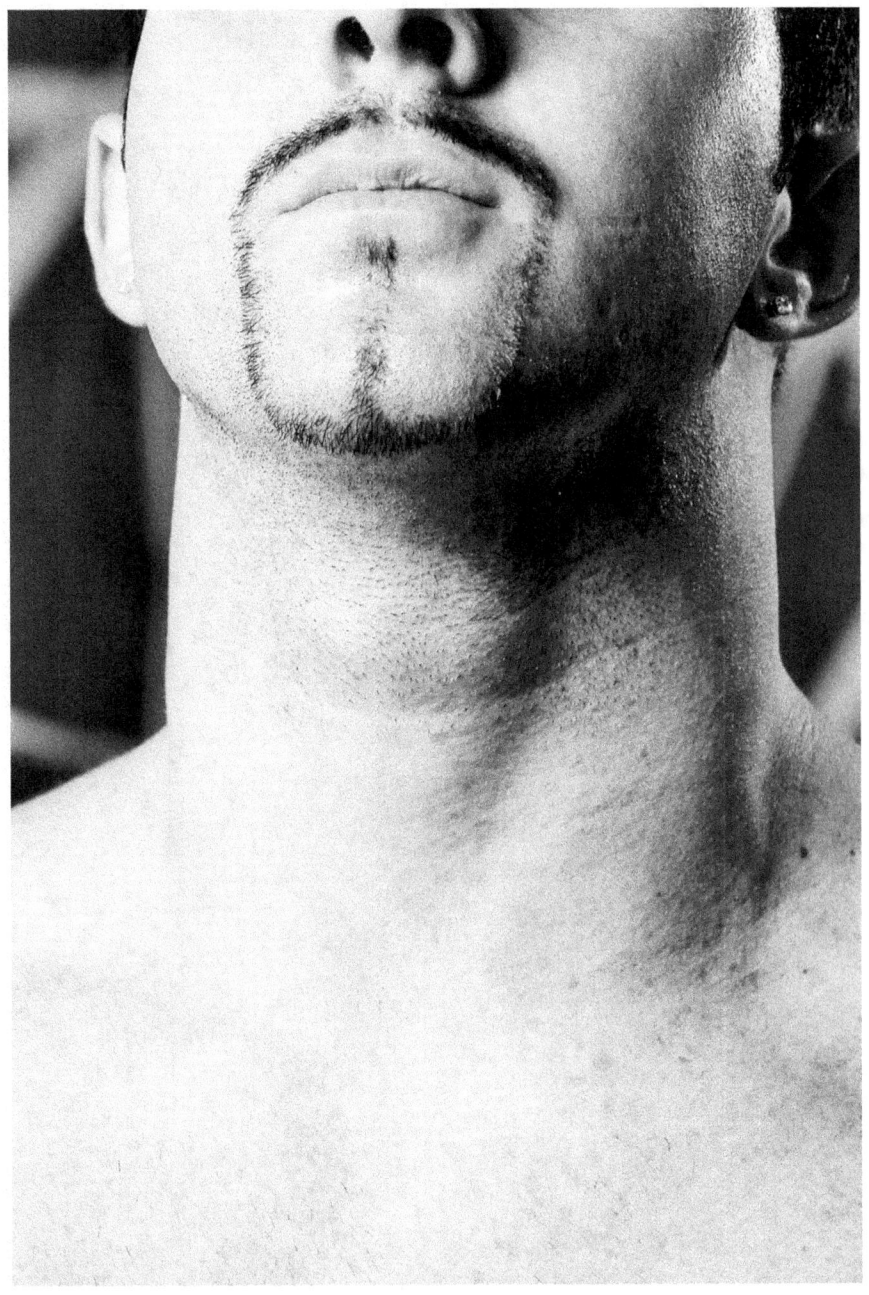

## irresponsible impregnation

Somewhere, down one of the main thoroughfares of the Kingdom, in an expansive house surrounding a courtyard, lives the spiritual player: the stereotypical playboy.

He is a type who loves and lives for the process of conquest, impregnation and conception, but at the end of the day is generally irresponsible with his impregnation: not planning for the vision he sires, leaving his multiplied children without adequate care or sustenance.

Enjoying the thrill of what he perceives to be the birthing of vision; he spreads the seed of his creative ideas all over the place.

In the process he is not discriminate like the farmer whose seed is sown in neat, even rows, planted with an eye towards the greatest harvest yield; but he is as one whose joy in life is not the success of the harvest to come but the immediately gratifying thrill of the act of casting as much seed as far a field as possible.

The fruit of the farmer's sowing in those neat rows of plowed earth is produce that can be weeded, watered and tended to until the hour of harvest; a harvest that will fill the barns with plenty to feed himself and his family through the long winter's chill. And he will have seed enough left over to replicate and multiply a similar harvest in the next season of sowing, and a sizeable portion to sell for cash or give to the needy.

The player's sowing is not as productive. Certainly one can make a valid point that seed sown far a field still produces spiritual babies. Our friend's sowing produces multiple children who spring up in a spontaneous fashion around the Kingdom.

It is the long-term effectiveness and sustainability of his children that is in question.

⊢————————————————⊣

It is only when we step off the street, enter the courtyard of his residence and take a closer look at the multiplied off-spring that bare his name we observe that they all appear to be in various states of arrested development.

Some of his children appear to be pre-toddlers, sitting at his feet, pulling on the cuffs of his slacks. A few are actually toddlers, waddling around him in a space of only a few feet from his imposing presence, falling down every few steps that are taken.

Noticing our interest in his offspring, he says that he has some older children, who he quickly ushers into the court-yard from their rooms on one side of the complex; but for their age, they look as small and indistinguishable from the rest.

And even the new-born visions, the most recent additions to his family, show the signs of beginning malnutrition: hollow cheeks, the extended belly and the pencil thin limbs that are seen in the children of draught and famine.

The Player is obviously proud of his offspring. Honorably, they all bare his family name, and he can energetically spout off the birth name that he gave each one of them: ministry, outreach, mission, program, strategy, school, institute; with impressive middle names like global, international, overcoming, conquerors, world-wide—names that belie the fact that his children are raggedy and half-starved.

Despite his already large brood—by now we have seen all from the youngest to the oldest visions—he energetically leaves our presence, returning a few minutes later with a couple new babies that he proudly displays for us before he sets them on the ground with their motley assortment of brothers and sisters.

No, these were not children that he already had when we entered his courtyard but forgot to bring out with the earlier group, but were new visions: ideas that he conceived during the short tenure of our interaction.

## the drug of choice

The unfortunate truth about our new friend, the Player, is that he is an addict.

His addiction is not that of so many who aimlessly wander the halls of the kingdoms of men, shooting, snorting or sniffing whatever will give them a momentary escape from a life that is either extremely mundane or too full of pain to be experienced with a clear head.

The drug of choice for our friend is the high he gets from the spiritual transaction that takes place when he plants the seed of his vision.

His high is a euphoria that when pursued never fails to raise his levels of spiritual testosterone and thyroid so that any lethargy is vanquished as he bounds with fresh energy and stamina.

In his state of vision-casting, he feels that he is most in tune with himself, the cosmos, and in his inaccurate belief, the Beloved. The only problem is that once the planting is done and the vision conceived, the drug-like euphoria that was such a welcome byproduct of his actions quickly dissipates.

For our new friend, we observe that the momentary spiritual high of casting the seed of vision eventually turns into a valley low, a deep dark place, where the player mopes and gropes until he realizes that he needs to actively search for his next fix.

It doesn't take him long to ponder the exhilaration that he received from the last seed planting, which sends him on a trek, looking for the next opportunity to cast vision into any available and receptive ground.

In the process of spreading the seed of vision to and fro in the Kingdom, the player doesn't realize that, even in what he may believe is the sincerity of his heart, he has in error subjugated the natural order: that the Beloved is the one who plants His seed in a willing womb vs. us spreading the seed that we have developed from a superior intellect and creative proclivities into the ground of others.

Fearing the depths of the emotional and spiritual valley—and not willing to have the patience or understanding of the process to walk through conception, the morning sickness and travail—it becomes too easy for our friend to recreate the "rush" he receives from planting seed with a miserable substitute of his own making that looks and sounds like vision but lacks the divine spark needed to germinate and produce a viable offspring.

---

The unfocused spreading of seed by our friend equates to a dissipation of energy and life. (Energy is multiplied when focused on the nurture and care of the seed that the Beloved plants in our womb.)

There is only so much energy that a person can have; only so much seed that a person can spread.  As seed is spread, energy is dissipated.

The Beloved waits in the sidelines for such a one to run out of energy and seed, experience the futility of and lack of fruit associated with his vision-casting, until he comes back to Him.

## don't plan for what you sire

The great tragedy for the spiritual player is three-fold: not only does he not understand that he is the one planting the seed, when his real role should as the one receiving the seed of purpose and vision from the beloved, he also doesn't plan for what he sires, nor does he care for what he conceives.

The spiritual player's main pleasure in life is conceiving new babies, but he has little time or focus for the weighty matters of planning for the birth, and nurture and development of the children he sires until the day they are able to stand on their own, or be passed to the responsibility of another.

If he understands his own limitations and brings into the picture those who can care for the children, there is a possibility that some may survive and even thrive.

But, unfortunately, it is a rare player that understands his need to be surrounded by the nannies and nursemaids: caretakers of the Kingdom's visions. He may see these key individuals as potentially stifling his freedom to do and say and be whatever he wants when he wants to!

When the caretakers begin to plan for the nurture and development of the vision, it means that there will be structure and accountability brought into the player's life.

It will be no longer acceptable that his children are in multiple stages of malnutrition or sitting in their own organizational excrement.

Without the caretakers at hand, he can continue to believe whatever he wants about the fruit of his loins. He can continue to see his success in the Kingdom in terms of the multiplicity of programs, corporations or entities that bare his name instead of their actual viability.

Sadly, our friend is like the king in the old story who was naked, yet believed that he had on some fine threads; but because of fear, none of his subjects would acknowledge that the king had no clothing.

A player without the structure and accountability brought by the caregivers is a deluded emperor without any raiment. He may think he has been successful, his people may say the same, but the ordinarily modestly covered body parts dangling out in full public view testify that he is buck naked!

Some spiritual players do come to the understanding that they are loose with their seed, their children often do not survive much past birth, and the few friends that hang out with them are run ragged attempting to keep up with the never ending process of following flung seed in an attempt to see it sprout; while the player almost immediately has wandered over to another corner of the Kingdom to continue the planting process.

Often the player is aware of their need for the caregivers but has only a limited tolerance for what they bring to his vision.

The issue again is that the player does not want to be accountable for the thing he sires. If he is accountable he has to admit occasional or complete defeat; rethink his plan of action and purpose in the Kingdom, and may need to admit that the Beloved has been left completely out of the birth process in his life and ministry.

He may even have to admit that his visions are a pale reflection of the Beloved's; owning up to the fact that he has not been experiencing spiritual intimacy with the Beloved but a form of spiritual masturbation: the stimulation of an overly active ego or intellect in the pursuit of self-gratifying activities that are not building the Kingdom, with a capital "K", but a lesser, and in reality pathetic kingdom, with a small case "k".

## don't care for what you conceive

Responsibility, Kingdom stewardship and common sense say that if you are not going to plan for what you sire or care for your conceptions that you should not be birthing any babies.

In the mind of the young teenage boy, he sees his ability to copulate as a sign of his masculine virility; yet as long as his ability to do so is not connected with the responsibility of his need to care for what he conceives, he has not moved to the place of maturity that is needed to be a parent.

If you are too young in the Kingdom or too immature to be responsible, you are better off waiting. In our context, the currently used, popular phrase, "true love waits" means that you will not create visions that are premature and only serve to promote your false sense of spiritual virility.

True love will subject all that is immature, that is of the self serving fleshy ego, to the beloved. And, over time will grow in intimacy to the same, and eventually find a womb swimming full of divine potential and purpose.

•——————————————————————•

If we do wait on the Beloved's timing and allow Him to plant the seed and work through our humility, we will find that He is the perfect Father.

The Beloved will never prove to be a deadbeat dad.

If He is the Father of a thing, you don't need to worry that the photo of your vision will appear on the back of a milk carton as a lost or missing child, or that His photo will be publicly displayed on a poster in the local post office due to abandonment, abuse or neglect to pay child support.

When God is the Father of a vision He will always prove faithful to care for his conception. That does not mean that, following delivery, you will not lift another finger in the child's care.

But it does mean that He will bring the nannies and nursemaids you need at the right time; he will make sure there is always money to buy the diapers, and formula, and toys and books and pay for the tuition and care for the development of your vision from birth all the way to maturity.

As the birth parent, you may have to write a grant to secure adequate formula, have a fundraising event to pay for future schooling tuition and books, or even ask other friends in the Kingdom for some help; but, the Beloved's favor will ensure that He has gone before you to prepare the hearts of those who He wants to come by your side to help take care of His precious vision.

---

The player's keen intellect and creative skill are only useful in the Kingdom when he submits them to the Beloved, waiting in His presence, growing in intimacy until the Beloved's seed is planted in his spiritual womb.

When the natural order is subjugated the children of the player will eventually catch up with him—as the Kingdom citizens realize that behind the impressive names are malnourished and untended visions that do not bear the charisma or the character that should attend a vision from the Beloved.

## child abandonment—babies on the doorstep

Unfortunately, for every healthy vision in the Kingdom there are a number of babies that are inevitably abandoned on the doorstep.

These are programs, ministries and outreaches that, unlike the children of the player, were birthed out of a genuine intimacy with the Beloved, carried to term and brought into the world—perhaps even with a hint of fanfare—only to find their opportunities for survival limited because they are left out in the cold.

A baby on the doorstep is not a bastard child; it is fully a vision.  It has the same plump freshness of every newborn, and in a parental desire that the child survive its abandonment may even have the child's name pinned to their blanket for easier identification.

As with every newborn, so much promise resides in the little bundle, so much potential to develop and grow and impact the nations. When you jab the new vision with your finger, you feel the elasticity of something that is prepared to expand in depth and influence.

The baby on the doorstep is not the same as the player's children, who are kept within his realm of influence, and displayed to show his prowess as a spiritual stud.

Unfortunately, the doorstep child is not wanted or found no longer useful to the purposes of the Kingdom leader who brought it forth.  Its uselessness is reflected in that there is no budget to feed it, nor are there any tender and helping administrative hands standing in the sidelines waiting to guide the child from their early years to maturity.

The baby on the doorstep starts out healthy and is even attended to by great enthusiasm among the people the child is birthed for, but due to a lack of responsibility on the part of its birth parent is quickly forgotten and laid outside, in the vain hope that some volunteer will pick it up and feed, clean and clothe the vision.

Unfortunately, there are a rare few in the Kingdom who will pick up a child that has been abandoned. Most reason that they have no time for that which their leader had no use for.

Babies left on the doorstep usually die. The Kingdom leader gets to the place where he doesn't know what to do with the little thing, and in his inability to draw the appropriate help the child needs, it quickly expires.

Something that started strong can within a matter of weeks or months be long forgotten, a distant memory, and amazingly not even leave a trace of embarrassment in the Kingdom because all traces of its existence were quickly erased.

---

Babies on the doorstep can be conceived from a number of motivations that focus more on the self-serving mind of the parent than on the greater Kingdom good.

False motives can take the form of the person who wants to get pregnant but doesn't want to get married or take the Father's name. In this "one night stand with Jesus" scenario, the intimacy with the Beloved was a feigned means to an end: pregnancy.

For this one the fruit of the womb will eventually prove too burdensome because the birth parent refuses to draw from the life of the Father.

Some people only want a welfare baby: a child that will be expressly used to lift offerings; sustaining the leader's lifestyle on the backs of the good citizens of the Kingdom. This one does not care for the success or failure of the vision, but for their own gain, eventually leaving the child outside to die when the pockets are full of lucre.

During a short season of usefulness the child opens the hearts of others to give but is unceremoniously discarded or replaced once the magic draw to the donor is no longer present.

A baby on the doorstep is the fruit of one who used the opportunity for intimacy with the Beloved for their own gain. Such is the realm of spiritual fornicators and adulterers, who have feigned intimacy with the Beloved and born His children; but as all other fornicators, were never really wed to Him or His purposes.

Sadly the fruit of intimacy is misused, abused and cast off once the desires of the parent have been met.

# test tube babies, cloning, abortion and false labor

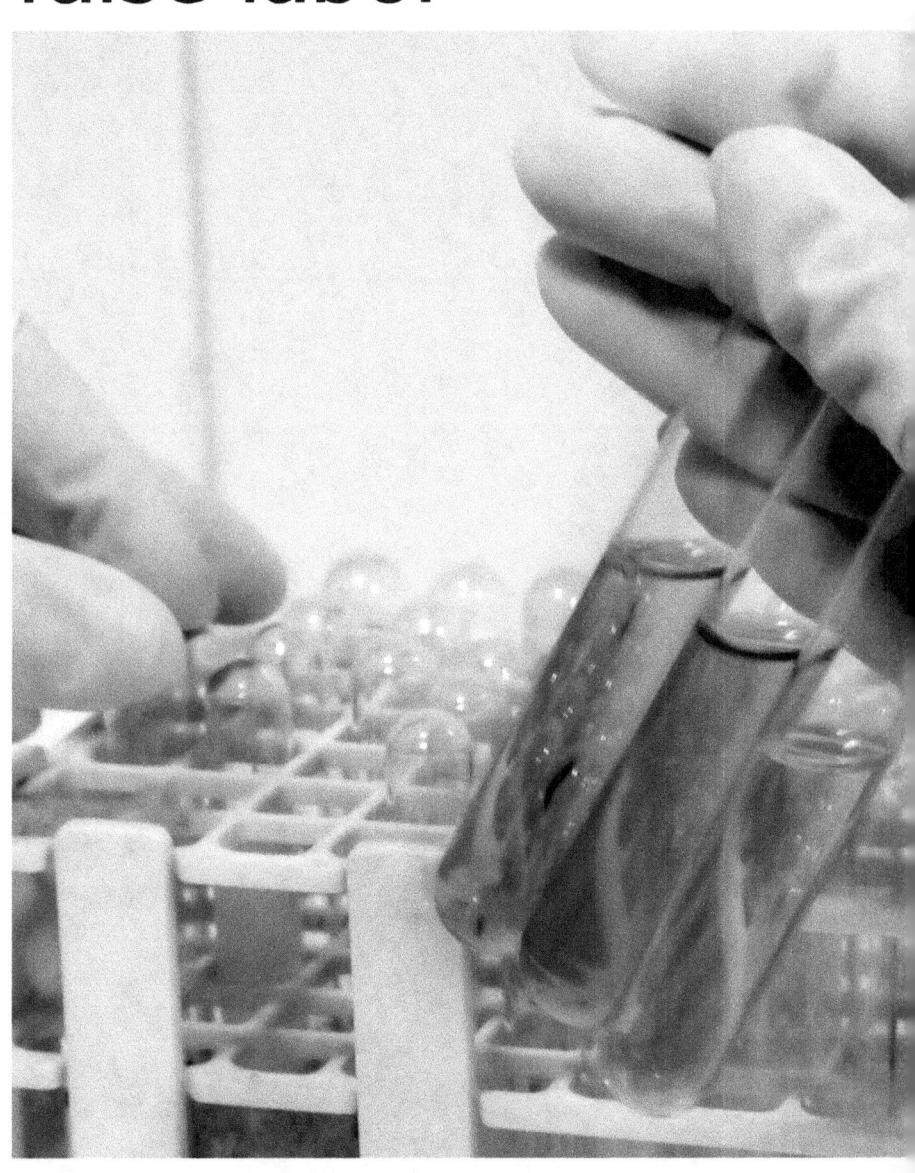

# test tube babies

The laboratory was a sterile environment. Great care was taken that all utensils were properly sanitized, and that the room was airtight: completely insulated from outside influences, with all incoming air filtered to ensure atmospheric purity.

The technicians, through years of research and trial and error, believed that they had distilled the Kingdom principle of birthing of vision down to its scientific and functional components.

Their aim was to find a way to create the life of a baby vision without all the uncomfortable months of carrying the vision, and the messy and agonizing travail and birthing process.

They believed that if they could isolate the seed of vision and recreate the reaction that takes place in the spiritual womb when purpose and power are planted—without all the other outside influences coming into play—that greater progress in the Kingdom could be made at less of a cost. And, that more people would be drawn toward their version of a less-uncomfortable Kingdom work.

With their rubberized medical gloves on; donning white surgical robes, hats and face masks they stood around a square box-like contraption that contained the fruit of years of experiments.

In it was approximately a dozen Petri dishes and a few test tubes filled with different murky gray substances. In one test tube they had successfully isolated the seed of purpose, separating it from the Seed-bearer.

One of the more studious in the bunch walked over to a blackboard at the end of the laboratory. Finding a piece of half-used chalk he began to scribble something on the board.

"Gentlemen and Ladies," he said, "the scientific equation for what we have just discovered can be summed up as following:

**{Seed of Purpose/Vision — Seed-bearer =
Power of Conception — Relationship/Intimacy}."**

His colleagues looked at each other in amazement. He had summed up in a few chalk scratches what they had spent countless months working to discover.

Once their awe over the scientific equation subsided they began to turn their attention back to the box-like contraption, focusing on a Petri dish used in their experiment to create their mechanical version of the spiritual womb.

They believed that, as they had isolated the seed from the Seed-bearer, they had as successfully recreated the components of proper temperature and nutrition that line a spiritual womb.

If successful, this breakthrough discovery would allow vision to be birthed and receive all the nutrients it needs to develop; but allow it to be nurtured in a dish in a temperature controlled environment instead of the conventional way: inside a living and breathing human being.

In the midst of their pondering the contents of the womb in a dish, the team members, almost in unison turned to their colleague who had so successfully summed up the earlier process into a scientific equation.

"How do you sum up this part of the experiment?" they asked.

"Very simply stated," was his reply, as he moved back toward the blackboard, erasing some other unnecessary equations to make room for his latest revelation. "This part of the equation can be summed up as

$$\{A\ Womb + Proper\ Nutrition - Humanity = A\ Cold\ Passionless\ Breeding\ Ground\}"$$

while the combination of the seed and womb together is summed up as

$$\{Power\ of\ Conception - Relationship/Intimacy + A\ Cold\ Passionless\ Breeding\ Ground = A\ Bast...\}.$$

As he came to the end of the final equation, the shock of what he was writing rattled his usually calm disposition causing the piece of chalk to fall out of the man's hand and on to the floor.

He and the group of his fellow colleagues stood in stunned silence, staring at the board.

The equations revealed significant flaws in the science that they had spent years working toward: it was not possible to create the life and potential of the Beloved in a sterile environment.

A vision birthed in an environment separate from intimacy and the passion of humanity was always something less than a true baby.

Even as the fruit of intimacy with the Beloved is always conception of a vision; so true is the converse: that there can be no baby without intimacy.

It is always in the humanity of men relating with the Divinity of the Father of the child that the heart of the vision is formed.

Once their shock subsided they realized that their years of experimentation were in vain.  It was not possible to create a vision imbued with Kingdom values and the life blood of the Beloved apart from relationship.

Science and religion told them that isolating the components of the process would allow them to manipulate the process.  But, without relationship and intimacy and a human womb, the potential product produced could not even be mentioned on the chalkboard.

## cloning

Even as a test tube baby is not appropriate as a birth in the Kingdom, likewise, the Kingdom is not a place for clones.

A clone is an exact DNA replica of an original template; it will look, smell and taste like the original but it is not, and never could take the place of the original.

As a Kingdom citizen you are destined to look like the

Beloved, but your organization and people do not need to look like you—nor do you need to look like the Kingdom leader down the street.

Producing a clone or a carbon copy of another in the Kingdom will only produce an empty cliché or a comical clown.

If you want to be a cliché/clown, you can clone a clown: simply wear the same style, color and cut of suit; brush and tint the hair in the same coiffeur and carry the same props. Then strut around the stage like the cheap imitation of greatness that you are attempting to be.

You may effectively copy mannerisms and methods, but you will always only ever be a clown.

The deception of Kingdom cloning is that the outward trappings that are represented in the clown and cliché can be cloned, but not the inner reservoir of character or charisma.

You can copy and recreate the ministry of a great man or woman of the Kingdom, you can even attempt to evoke the essence of the atmosphere that surrounds their presence, but you can never clone their character or charisma.

The Beloved's presence and favor rest where there is character. Where He is not the father of a vision it will lack the core of character and charisma that are the stamp of Kingdom vision.

Kingdom cloning divides off a form and façade of the ministry, program or outreach being imitated, but will inevitably leave the essence of the thing behind in the original.

The original may be a wonderful model, but it will never be replicated in power and purpose without the freshness that comes from taking it back to the Beloved, laying it in His presence, and on His approval allowing Him to implant the vision in your spiritual womb as He did to the original parent.

The key is to allow Him the right to be the father of a thing, even if it is a model that is already used to great success in other corners of the Kingdom's corridors.

Your baby may have grown to great significance and increase in numbers, finance and social and political influence, but that does not necessitate that my replicating your vision in my corner of the world will bring about the results that you have experienced.

Movements that begin in and of the Spirit, once copied in the outward form, in time become only shadows of the initial greatness when the vision is not birthed.

Character and charisma are produced in only one manner: they are birthed in one's life through the trials and pressure of the process.

There is no easy way to imitate character when the child was not carried in a womb through travail, and birthed in pressure.

There is a sort of lifeless, listless, empty charisma exhibited when a child does not have a genuine experience and testimony of making it through the warfare and agony that attended its nativity.

## abortion

The Kingdom leader had too much: too much disappointment, too much resistance, too much of the political maneuvering and power plays that left one feeling like a piece of flesh freshly pressed through an old fashioned meat grinder.

He was tired of Kingdom people and pursuits; but most of all was weary of carrying the Beloved's babies, tired of being barefoot and pregnant for Jesus.

The visions over the years that he conceived and carried in his womb, and the resultant birthing process had been costly: apparent damage had been done to the birth parent— the visions over the years had resulted, among other things, in a loss of relationships, a strain on financial security, a loss of weight and a challenge to his health; and seasons of looking just plain crazy to the other folks in the Kingdom.

In his wearied reasoning he just wanted some time and space for himself; not merely a season of sabbatical refreshment and retooling for a future of more births, but the ability to control the process, and establish his schedule and timeline for when he would be available to carry a vision to term.

Instead of evaluating his stewarding of the process of birth and effectiveness in delegating care for new children to allow for smoother future visions, his mindset told him that true freedom would only be found in his choosing which conceptions to retain.

His distressed thinking took him to a well-polished storefront on the edge of a kingdom beyond the boundary of the Beloved's over in that of men: **The Family Planning Center**, whose motto: "*We will help you have controlled fulfillment of your vision and purpose without infringing on your personal life*" was emblazoned across the front of the welcome desk.

Upon entering the clinic, a smiling receptionist motioned him to an empty chair, handing him some free literature to read while he waited for his appointment. One brightly colored pamphlet carried a message about the role of the diaphragm and prophylactic in blocking the seed of purpose from the spiritual womb; concluding that if disobedience and pride did not stop the seed there were still other options...

A second pamphlet spoke of the audacity and unfairness of a deity that did not practice spiritual birth control, and whose presence always resulted in pregnancy, despite the withered deadness of the womb or the advancement in age or the medical improbability of a birth taking place. How could one deemed so beloved be trusted when He alone controlled the timing and frequency of the planting of the seeds of vision and purpose?

As he finished the last pamphlet the nice receptionist drew his attention to a television monitor across the room. The video presentation opened with an idyllic scene of a leader like him dancing through a lush green field.

The narration began: "Don't you deserve your space and to be able to taste the sweetness of the reward of your service? Didn't you already birth and run those other visions? Aren't there enough babies running around the globe without you adding any more to the congested avenues of the King dom?"

The leader pulled away from the narrative on the screen to the monologue in his mind.  He had struggled too long for the sake of the Kingdom, and too long had reckoned himself a servant of the Beloved.

He didn't want any more babies until he decided.  No more carrying something that the Beloved planted in his womb, but was not in his best interests.

He reasoned further that his desire to abort the seed of vision was not just an issue of inconvenience, an excuse many in the Kingdom had used; but his was a justified medical crisis, and the conception in his womb could potentially cause his death if carried to full term.

## the fruit of aborted vision

The physical womb of a woman should be the most protected place in the universe.  In it a child is conceived, nourished and shielded from harm; with hopefully all the focus and attention of the mother being paid to the needs of the precious cargo she carries.

In reality it is sadly not so.  The procedure to abort a baby is considered common and clinical; with a child more likely to be killed before ever exiting the womb than he/she might be through disaster, famine or terror attacks on this side of the womb.

Many modern Kingdom citizens like to control the number of spiritual children they have and when they have them; and when it is inconvenient for their modern life, they will abort.

Spiritual abortion is a scraping away, sucking out and discarding of that which God has placed in one's spiritual womb. It is a disregard of the thing within that Mary spoke of as holy, so that the convenience of the moment eclipses the desire of the Kingdom.

The result of a spiritual abortion is a vacant place in

one's belly. Where formerly there was life: potential and promise wrestling with each other, like twins, to see who the greatest part of the vision was; there is now only emptiness: a cold,cavernous place.

The fruit of the abortion is a deep feeling of dislocation from life, and a vulnerability to a wide range of emotions from depression, sorrow, and despair.

---

There are three responses from one who has aborted the vision of God: One, a jaded numbness to the things of the Kingdom.

When one makes the eventual realization that they are enveloped with deadness with what should have been a season of great joy—the shock of what they have done is too great to carry, and they pull back into a place of vacant stares whenever the work or words of the Beloved are spoken.

The second response is a self-denial that one was ever pregnant with God's vision, or that one ever understood the purposes of God in spiritual pregnancy.

The one in self denial is like Prissy, the house slave in antebellum Tara, who once touted that she knew everything about birthing babies. Yet, in the hour of travail she cried, "I don't know nothin' about birthing no babies, Miss Scarlet!"

The third response is a realization that what had been planted in the womb actually was a holy thing from the Beloved; and in making light of the holy, one discarded in a dumpster the purposes that He had intended you to carry.

The third response is by far the most painful. While the other two responses leave one numbed or wrapped in denial and in a broken relationship with the Beloved; the third acknowledges and brings the guilt, shame and agony of the aborted vision back to Him, who alone can forgive, heal and restore.

The leader's attention was jerked from his internal monologue to the sterile waiting room by the voice of the smiling receptionist.

"Sir," she said, "the doctor will see you now.

Go through the door, turn left, and enter the first room on the right. The doctor will be right in, perform the procedure and we will have you back to afternoon activities in a few minutes."

The leader put the colorful pamphlets on the waiting room coffee table, picked up his cell phone and walked through the door...

## false labor

There was nothing there. After the weeks and months of walking around like one pregnant with vision and purpose, at the end of the day there was no breaking of water, no delivery and no baby.

Only a moment separated between the feeling of a full womb, and an expectant hope that a birth was imminent and the current state of burst expectations. The thing that looked so much like a child of promise was nothing but an empty dream.

The Kingdom Citizen looked at herself in the full-length mirror. The slight bags under her eyes were a reflection of the emotional weariness that she felt in her soul.

She thought she had walked with the Beloved for enough years to know when the seed of vision was planted in her spiritual womb. In fact, she recalled the hour that she felt the spark of life ignite her spirit. From that moment forward she was so certain that she was with child.

The excitement over being chosen by the Beloved had bubbled up during the months of waiting and carrying what she thought was a baby vision.

Her friends even commented that she was already talking like the expected end had come; that mentally and emotionally she was behaving like a mother in the Kingdom.

The Kingdom citizen turned from the mirror, shuffled over to the sofa on the opposite side of the room; grabbed her belly and cupped it with both hands.

She had certainly known such a wonderful intimacy with the Beloved over the months, combined with what she thought were birthing pangs; even some long nights of prayer where her soul was vexed by the enemy of her soul to disbelieve the character and beneficence of the Beloved in her life.

She even had a couple nights where the dark enemy bade her to abandon the pregnancy that she thought she was carrying.

The sad realization faced her today that she had been through the motions of a pregnancy; had believed that there was a vision to be birthed, but in the end that there was no baby.

Her heart ached. She wanted to cry but knew if she allowed herself even a moment of grief it would lead her down a slope of despair that she could not quickly recover from.

Where yesterday she was praying into—spiritually and emotionally leaning forward into her future—today she was only a combination of numbness and sharp pain.

---

It was as if she had over the weeks climbed the rungs of a ladder of expectation, up one level, then another, until she reached the pinnacle: the top of a high diving board.

Once at the top, she ignored the altitude, her inner fear of heights, the narrowness of the board, and moved to the edge in faith knowing that the Beloved was with her.

Once at the edge she poised herself with the grace of the Olympic trained: hands over her head, leaning forward, and jumped from the board only to find out that the pool was not filled with water.

The shock and the pain were that real to her mind and heart. She never knew that outside of the death of a loved one, one could hurt so much.

Of course, in reality, this was the death of a loved one; what she thought was a vision that was planted in her womb, that she grew to cherish and long for the expectant day when she could push forth and display that which the Beloved had done for her.

---

Our Kingdom Citizen wrestled with the question of "why" for months.  Why had this happened?

Perhaps she had not laid a fertile enough ground of prayer and the baby never really connected to the moist lining of the nutritious place; perhaps the vision had died weeks ago, and in her strong desire to bare the Beloved's child, she had deluded herself that a dead space was still full of life—a sort of hope against hope situation where the heart wants to believe the impossible even when all signs point to the opposite.

Or perhaps she had never really been pregnant!  In her strong desire to birth had she misinterpreted the spiritual signs, that the intimacy with the Beloved was for her own nurture and healing and had nothing, at least in her present state, to do with pregnancy?

Had she then strung together circumstances, playing out a role of recipient in what she thought was a string of divine interventions...what was in actuality coming to false conclusions about mere coincidence.

She didn't know what the answer was, but knew that she was empty, hurt and felt a deep cavernous vacant space in her inside that longed to be touched by His tender hand.

Now reclined on her sofa, tucked under the cover of an old frayed but warm afghan, she rolled over on her side and faintly whispered a prayer, not prompted by one with a full and overflowing inner self, but simply the numb words of an aching and empty heart.

# will I conceive again?

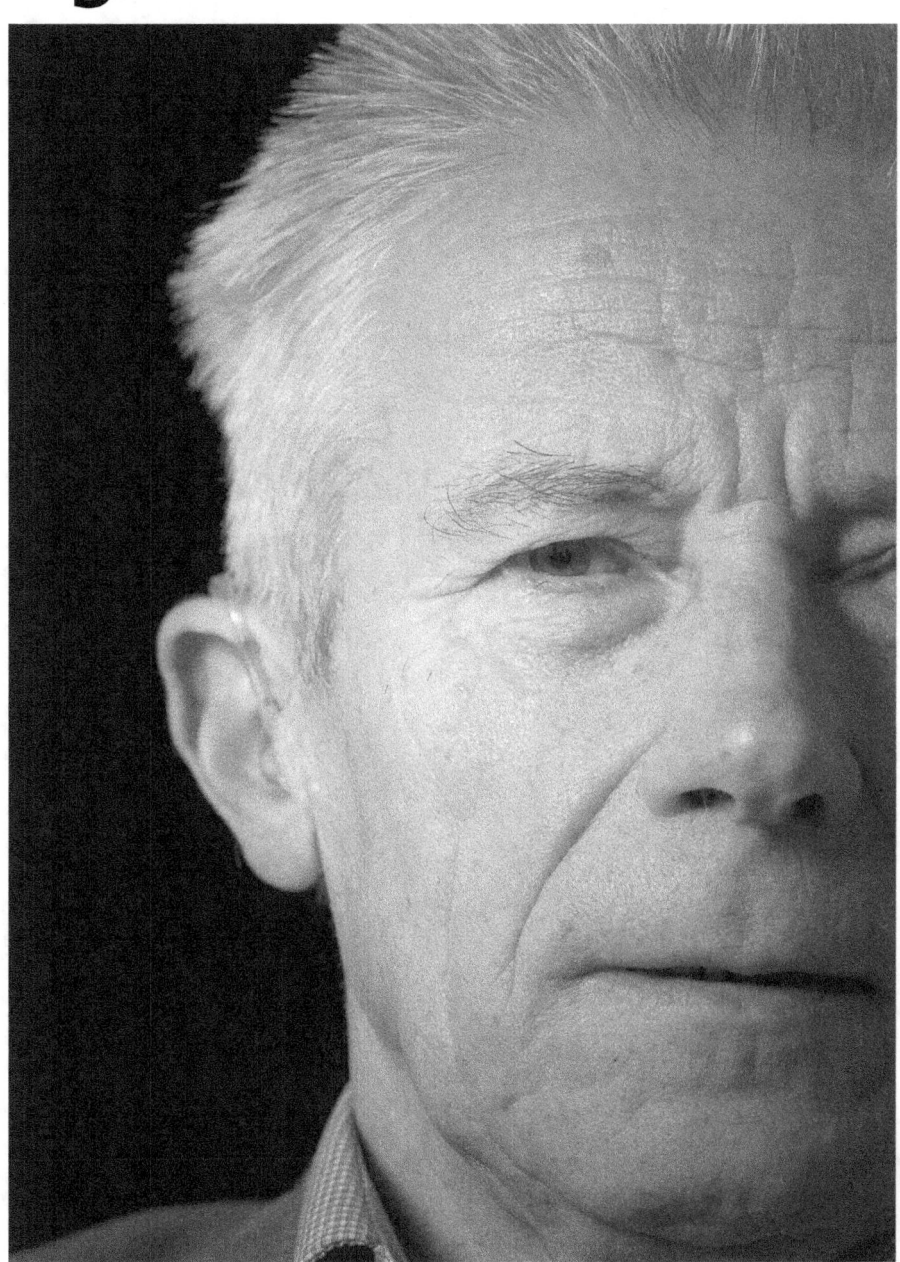

## abraham and sarah

Abraham and Sarah were biologically too old to be parents. Sarah's womb was all dried up; and her equally old husband had a feeble and slow, if not totally used up sperm bank—an account that had long experienced its final transaction; had run out—account closed!

Even if Abraham still had some life in his procreative functions, and a lone sperm traversed the journey to Sarah's womb; there was nothing there to greet it at the end of the trip.

The issue of the lifeless reproductive organs of this patriarchal couple becoming the place of conception for a child was a miracle, and a predominant focus of the exposition of the texts in the Abraham and Sarah narrative.

It was a miracle unattested in that biology, human physiology and agrarian common sense would say that there was no possible way that fertility could spring from infertility.

Yet somehow the Beloved's promise was made to this elderly couple—a promise with historical ramifications that would go way beyond their small, middle-east desert, sphere of influence and mentality—a promise that would produce a people that through time would testify to the Beloved's faithfulness and care.

The baby birthed from the womb of Sarah was a son: Isaac, the child of promise who would multiply and carry on the seed and covenant of the Beloved made to Abraham for the nations.

The Beloved had showed Himself faithful to His promise by choosing the favored way of His provision: taking a dried up barren womb and birthing a baby.

**The Beloved delights in getting the glory from bringing life to dead places and spaces.**

The issue with conception of spiritual vision never rests on the barrenness of the womb God chooses. It matters not to Him that in biblical language the couple is well stricken with years.

Their inability in the flesh to produce offspring does not negate the promise of God.  In fact, it actually confirms the promise being from Him, as the parents are unable in themselves to create life.

The seed of the vision always originates from God and the miracle of the chosen vessel He uses is His doing.

There is no retirement in Kingdom business.  If we are truly submitted to Him and His will, and continue to cultivate our relationship of intimacy with the Beloved well into our senior years, and we refuse contraception; there will always be conception and new babies born.

Attitude, not age is the only factor that will stop us from being birth parents for the vision of God. Kingdom fertility is God's business, ours is a willingness to be His vessel and have Him do unto us as He desires.

Even when the hair is gray and the eyesight is growing dim, the prayer of our heart should still be that of the young virgin that we are the handmaiden of the Lord—albeit a wrinkled and bent version—and that He can still do unto us as He pleases.

The excuses of age, weariness and slowness of movement, while very real, are not hindrances to the aged one whose heart is yet inclined towards Him.

# a low libido

Beyond the miraculous conception and birth was what was unspoken in the text: that Abraham and Sarah were the age of most great-grandparents, having to raise an energetic bundle of new life.

The recorded miracle is the conception and birth of Isaac, but the greater miracle might be the one that we never talk about: how the elderly parent's energy level held up once the little baby came on the scene.

Certainly, Abraham and Sarah were wealthy enough to have nursemaids, nannies and other servants.  But, even with the help, the Parent's limited energy and attention were likely always focused on this their God-given heir.

How many nights did Sarah hobble around the tent, wringing her boney hands with concern over Isaac's fever and cough? How long could Abraham play games in the sand with his growing son before the old man had to lie down for a rest?

---

Somehow God ordained that physical childbearing would be the most fruitful for adults from their late teens to their early thirties. The sperm count is highest, the eggs the most fertile and the sex drive the greatest.

The people who birth babies during this fertile period will be dealing with the late nights of infancy and the rambunctious toddler and early school years with the energy level of a twenty- to fifty-ish something; not that of a nonagenarian or centenarian.

For the older parent who conceives, their child's increasing energy levels will be in direct contrast to their decreasing energy levels.

For the older spiritual birth parent the same holds true. The newborn vision of one's old age will be no different than those of one's youth, requiring the same investment in attention and energy.

No matter the age of the parent, the baby vision will need to be feed, cleaned, disciplined and exercised to survive.

The older birth parent will need to accommodate for their lower energy level by drawing in caretakers who have the energy to run with and facilitate the new vision.

If you understand your limitations, that you can't put in the hours of work you once could, that you can't move as fast or as far and your memory is not the sharp detailed machine as it was when you were a youth; pace yourself and find some hard-working, fast moving and mentally sharp nannies to catch the baby you birth and see that it gets what it needs to thrive.

In the Kingdom of the Beloved, old age is never an excuse to close up one's spiritual womb.

As long as the Beloved has a will and purpose to establish among humankind, and while you still have breath in your lungs, blood flowing through your veins, are in your right mind and have a heart that beats in rhythm to His; He has babies for you to birth.

## noah the senior citizen

*"But Noah found favor in the eyes of Jehovah ...Noah was a righteous man, (and) perfect in his generations: Noah walked with God"* (Gen 6:8-9)

Noah was the prediluvian patriarch whose obedience to Jehovah provided the means for the survival of the human race and families of animals in the midst of the destruction of all life on earth.

In a world that had turned its back on Jehovah and walked in great wickedness and rebellion, Noah was righteous, perfect in his generation and he walked with God.

As one who was on intimate terms with the Beloved, He became fertile ground in which the Beloved could plant the seed of vision.

For Noah, the baby was an ark: a large wooden vessel that would float in water.

Noah's labor was long and hard, daily making manifest the child of promise that the Beloved had called him alone to carry to term; hauling wood, preparing the wood for lumber, forming the ark plank by plank, adding pitch to seal up the lumber—all in a desert region, with no major body of water nearby, a baby conceived and born to a world that had never seen rain from the sky, nonetheless a devastating flood the likes of what Noah described.

For decades Noah birthed that baby, laboring despite the mocking of crowds and the doubts of sanity by his family and friends; his labor and message of coming destruction ignored by a generation that despised the word and presence of the Ancient of Days.

His baby was humongous, the affect on the then known world unrivaled, and when the time of delivery was nigh, the breaking of the water that signaled the final hours of travail flooded the land, causing his child to float to its destiny.

---

In the midst of an age where men lived centuries instead of mere decades, Noah was a senior among the senior citizens.

As a late bloomer, Noah fathered his three sons around the age of 500 when most others in the biblical account fathered their children between a youthful 65 to 187 years.

As an older parent Noah only had three sons and their wives to fill the limited space in the ark vs. multiple generations that would have been produced had he sired in his youth.

Parallel to the birth of his sons, the seed of vision for the ark was planted early in Noah's 500's and completed at approximately 600 years of age.

At an age when his peers were basking in the fruit of their loins, surrounded by generations of grand, great and great-great grandchildren, Noah and wife were raising their first offspring.

In a season of life when others spent their hours sitting at the village gate discussing the events of the day; Noah labored to birth a big baby.

Noah was an old man, intimate with the Beloved, called to carry the seed of a world-preserving vision—and he was found faithful as a birth-parent.

The Beloved primarily looks for the heart that is inclined toward Him—not merely the date of birth, or stage in life. He bypassed all the younger, stronger men of the day for an old man who loved His presence and had a receptive spiritual womb that would carry the Beloved's child to term.

Noah was so much in love that he was willing to look crazy in the eyes of his neighbors. His message was not understood nor appreciated, and his name and reputation likely became a joke among his peers.

The vindication of the parent and his child took place when Noah's family and the menagerie of the animal kingdom entered the ark, the door was sealed and in the midst of the wailing of dying humanity, the big baby fulfilled its purpose: to preserve a remnant of those in whom Jehovah had breathed the breath of life.

## God can do it again!

Here I am in an intimate night again, years later. Although my flesh is a bit more wrinkled and in places hangs on my frame, my spiritual ground is still elastic and firm.

Although the Beloved now speaks to me in the dreams of the fathers—because I sleep more—vs. the visions of youth, the process is still the same. Familiarity in my relationship with Him breeds intimacy, and intimacy always results in a womb impregnated with the seed of vision, purpose and destiny.

I can't bend my legs in prayer like I used to; my knees resist the hard floor and after some time in the same position, I find myself unable to easily rise again and straighten up without difficulty.

But, even so, my heart still bends in solemn reverence before the One who has been my lover for so many stages and ages of life.

I can no longer run with the youth, but my lips can still speak His name and my heart yet beats quickly when His presence is made real to me.

"*I once was young, but now am old...*" yet I know that His time for me will not be complete until I have brought forth all the purpose and vision that He intends for me to birth.

"*...I have never seen the righteous forsaken or their seed begging bread*" (Ps 37:25). I know that if He chooses to impregnate me in my middle or latter years that He will provide that which is needed to care for His seed.

The child of my older years will correspond to that which I am able to carry and care for. As it was in my youth, the Beloved will not give me something that I am not equipped, or do not have the help to nurture and raise.

I realize though, that the energy level required of a fresh vision will challenge and inspire me to move with a new vigor.

But, the simple knowledge that the Beloved is not done with His servant is enough to make me run with the focus and energy of a much younger Kingdom denizen.

Knowing that He still has purpose and destiny for me, even when so many from the kingdom of men believe one should slow down or retire is enough motivation for me to open my womb to the seed of vision.

---

As I sit in my recliner, I recall the earlier children that I birthed; many now well-matured in their years and stature in the community. Programs and organizations that have touched countless generations of Kingdom seekers and citizens; many that have progressed through numerous caregiver's hands until I really didn't know who was walking at the side of the mature vision.

Leaning on the arm of the overstuffed chair I reached for a small black book on the end table at its side—it was my book of contacts of fellow sojourners from the years past.

Thumbing through the dog-eared, yellowed pages, I came to the name of my former nanny. I wondered what she'd been doing in recent years. I had seen her photos in some philanthropy publications and heard rumors of the visions she had helped to grow.

It was a long-shot that I had nanny's correct contact information, but even so I reached over for the black, rotary dial phone that sat next to the now open small black book.

Pulling the heavy cloth covered cord from behind the

table legs, I plopped the phone up on my lap, took my forefinger and dialed the number... "Ring, ring, ring"...went the phone; and again, "Ring, ring, ring".

I heard the receiver click, and a mature sounding older woman said, "This is nanny, how may I help you?"

"Nanny!" I gleefully shouted, almost jumping up off the overstuffed chair. "Nanny, is that really you?"

"I know who I am, but who are you?" she curtly replied.

"It's your old friend, Kingdom Citizen," said I.

Recognizing me, her voice seemed to light up over the phone as she somehow became less of a middle-aged woman, and more of the young one that I knew so many years before.

Nanny and I talked for hours, telling of our adventures over the years with the Beloved, sharing a tear over His faithfulness to us through many trials, and laughing together over stories of bungled missions past and our amazing human frailty.

As the conversation seemed to be naturally coming to a close with a pause in the reminiscence and banter, I asked a question: "Nanny, are you ready to do it again?"

She responded by asking what I meant, but immediately started talking about the pain in her legs, and the swelling in her hands, and the 'plus-two' level reading classes that now graced her face on a daily basis.

When she finished with her litany of complaint, I asked her once more: "Nanny, are you ready to do it again?"

This time the response to my question was a dead silence over the phone for what seemed like minutes. Then out of the silence she responded to me with another question: "What! Are you pregnant again?"

We both started laughing, I at her sharp wit and tongue, she at the obvious delight I took to her question.

As the long and hearty laughter died down, with the giddiness and verbal glow of one freshly impregnated with purpose, vision and destiny I began to recall my most recent experience of the Beloved wooing me, and the fresh sense of His presence and weight of His glory in my room and life.

"I believe I am once again pregnant," I stated. "I don't know fully what the child will look like, or how it will be cared for, but I know that I know that my womb is full, and my heart once again sings for joy at being chosen as a vessel fit for His use! To be honest, I was beginning to feel like I was all used up in the Beloved's service, but I now know differently."

"How far along are you?" Nanny questioned.

"Oh, a couple months," I replied. "I've been up every night the past few weeks between three and four in the morning, praying and writing down the plans and structure as the Beloved shares it with me; I can feel the vision kicking on the inside—I think it's a big baby this time!"

"Oh-my!" Nanny exclaimed. "You know I've gotten awards over the years for the way I lay out a nursery and set a feeding schedule, and the old pram is up in the attic—and there are some young Kingdom Citizens that I have been mentoring who can execute all the details for us and learn the process of birthing and caring for a vision."

By the time we hung up the phone, it was all planned—nanny was willing and ready to establish yet another award-winning nursery; and here I was, in my middle years, once again pregnant with fresh purpose: a Kingdom vision gestating and growing in my spiritual womb.

———————————————————

As I sat in the silence of my thoughts, I felt a familiar presence in the room: it was the Beloved.

I put the phone on the end table, raised my now free hands in the air and opened my lips to speak His name.

Praise and tears flowed from the lips and ducts of one who was full and grateful—from that night, so many years ago, where my heart was broken and eyes moist with the pain of loss over the child that had been taken from my side, to new vision and fresh pregnancy with Kingdom purpose—He had proven Himself faithful—God had done it again!

# questions

1. Do you have a relationship with the Beloved?

2. Is intimacy with Him a strong desire?

3. Is your spiritual womb open to His presence and touch?

4. Have you removed all forms of spiritual birth control disobedience and pride—from your life?

5. Are you ready to be pregnant with and carry to term the Kingdom purpose that He has for your life?

*If you answered yes to all the above questions, I pray two things:*

**One,** that the eyes of your heart would be enlightened so that you may know the hope to which he has called you (Eph 1:18)

**And, two,** that he would make all grace abound to you, so that in all things at all times, having all that you need, you will abound in every good work (2 Cor 9:8-9).

**The understanding of His purposes and the provision to fulfill those purposes will ensure fruitfulness as you birth Kingdom Vision.**

# contact the author for:

## speaking
Training Seminars
Motivational Teaching
Biblical Preaching

## life coaching
Assessment of where you are in the birthing process
Assessment of what is needed to carry to term
A mid-wife to help you birth your vision

## organizational development consultation
Strategic Planning
Organizational Structural Development
Establishment of a Kingdom Nursery to care for your vision

## writing
Creative Writing
Editorial Comment
Literary Coaching

Yeazell Consulting
P.O. Box 383194
Duncanville, Texas  75138
info@yeazellconsulting.com

## Tell us what you think of "The Baby".
comments@thebaby-site.com

## To order additional copies of this book go to:
www.thebaby-site.com
www.amazon.com

BookSurge, LLC
www.booksurge.com
1-866-308-6235
orders@booksurge.com

www.ingramcontent.com/pod-product-compliance
Lightning Source LLC
Chambersburg PA
CBHW060521290526

45791CB00001B/474